HOW TO
RELIEVE CRAMPS
AND OTHER
MENSTRUAL PROBLEMS

HOW TO RELIEVE CRAMPS
AND OTHER
MENSTRUAL PROBLEMS

—

Marcia Storch, M.D.
with Carrie Carmichael

WORKMAN PUBLISHING, NEW YORK

Library of Congress Cataloging in Publications Data

Storch, Marcia L.
How to relieve cramps and other menstrual
problems.
Includes index.
1. Menstruation disorders. I. Carmichael,
Carrie
II. Title.
RG161.S76   618.1'72   81-40508
ISBN 0-89480-191-0 (pbk.)   AACR2

Cover and book design: Geoffrey Stevens

Front cover photo: FPG-Zimmerman
Exercise illustrations: Sheila Camera

Workman Publishing
1 West 39 Street
New York, N.Y. 10018

Manufactured in the United States of America
First printing August 1982

10   9   8   7   6   5   4   3   2   1

To all the children:
Cara and Antoine Storch-Venghiattis
and
Casey and David Carmichael Greenfield

Marcia Storch
Carrie Carmichael

CONTENTS

CHAPTER ONE

THE CURSE NO MORE

In the beginning there was no menstruation in the Garden of Eden. Eve seems to have been created from Adam's rib without the need or ability to menstruate every month. But once she was seduced by the serpent into eating the apple (we assume it was red), she was banished from the Garden of Eden, doomed to painful childbirth and cursed—monthly. We are told that Eve, filled with shame, covered her nakedness. We are never informed as to what Eve wore during her periods—a diaper, napkin, tampon, double-strength fig leaf, or nothing at all. But other books of the Old Testament make it abundantly clear that the ability to menstruate was considered an extremely undesirable quality.

Menstruation has generally terrified most male-dominated societies. Monthly bleeding in the mature and maturing female, which starts and stops without illness, scarring, or intervention, can be mysterious and intimidating. Until the time of menopause, pregnancy—another magical condition—is basically the only thing that can make menstruation stop for any length of time, although the cycle is sometimes influenced by environmental stress, sickness, or drugs, all of which will be discussed later.

The primitive male often believed that the menstruating female radiated a threatening supernatural power, or *mana*. Because men could neither understand menstruation nor control it, they created elaborate rituals to keep themselves a safe distance from menstrual blood when they ate, hunted, and slept. Since a menstruating woman could not separate herself from her own blood, however, she became taboo. Many primitive cultures banished menstruating women from their tribes for four or five days every month. These women had to remove themselves to a menstrual hut set away from the community, and were

Some societies treated menstruation with fear and dread.

forbidden to mingle with both men and untainted women. Some were required to ritually purify themselves; others, luckier, were simply allowed to enjoy the solitude. One harassed woman of my acquaintance recently suggested that we bring back the custom. Even if a woman couldn't afford a room of her own, she would at least get a couple of days a month off.

Other primitive cultures were more extreme. The Carrier Indians in British Columbia made a newly menstruating girl live alone for as long as three or four years. She was forced to remain in the wilderness and to keep clear of any traveled paths she might defile. Some tribes in Cambodia forced their young maidens into seclusion for as long as three years. Since they were considered to be "in the shade," these women were not allowed to see the sun for the entire time they were set apart. Other Cambodian tribes required a hundred-day confinement, this in a bed under mosquito netting.

It is not clear what was supposed to go on while a woman was sequestered. Isolation certainly didn't stop a healthy female from menstruating when she rejoined society. However, when a young woman returned to her community, she was usually considered to be of marriageable age; with the absence of birth control in those days, her subsequent almost constant state of pregnancy would minimize further problems.

When a menstruating woman was allowed to mingle with others, she was forced to make her condition extremely obvious. She either had to scream out a warning to anyone who came near, wear a distinctive menstrual hat, or keep her eyes downcast.

These rituals and customs persist in primitive cultures today. The Mae Enga tribespeople in New Guinea believe that physical contact with either a menstruating woman or menstrual blood means slow death for a man. According to legend, after such contact he will vomit continuously, his blood will turn black, and his skin will darken and hang in folds. His mind will then go, and he will slowly drift ward death. One tribesman bserved by anthropologists in ie early 1960s divorced his wife or sleeping on his blanket while he had her period. Later, to make sure she couldn't infect him with sickness and evil, he killed er with an ax.

Not only primitive but some ighly advanced ancient cultures persecuted women because they menstruate. The Romans believed that physical ontact with a menstruating woman would cause trouble. The oman historian, Pliny, described the powers of these women in his *Natural History*. They were said to turn new wine our and make seeds dry up in ardens, to make fruit fall from ees and hives of bees die. These women were also supposed to ull the sheen of ivory and the dge of steel, dangerous for a oldier going into battle. Even ronze and iron were instantly lagued by rust when menstruating women were near.

Such prejudices did not die with the Roman Empire. During he 1920s, women believed a ermanent wave wouldn't take when a woman was menstruating. There still exists a folk belief n France that a woman can't make curdle-free mayonnaise at hat time of the month. Even hose of us who feel free of men-

strual taboos may carry a residual few. If you don't walk under ladders because you consider them unlucky, you have inherited your superstition from primitives who wouldn't pass under a bridge, tree, or clothesline when a menstruating woman was near to ensure that no dreaded blood or mana would fall on them.

Menstruation was not always frowned upon, however. Just as some societies treated menstruation with fear and dread, others felt that this awesome phenomenon, experienced only by women and uncontrollable by any man, had some magical medicinal powers. Leprosy was reported cured by menstrual blood, and warts and birthmarks erased. Conditions of goiter, gout, hemorrhoids, worms, epilepsy, and headaches improved. And, during the Middle Ages the menstrual blood of a virgin was supposedly most powerful: a virgin's first napkin was saved as a cure for the plague. Given the state of health in the Middle Ages, we can assume it did little good.

Roots of the Misunderstanding

The attitude toward menstruation recorded in the Old Testament has probably had a more direct effect on how women and men in the Judeo-Christian culture think about women's natural functions than did primitive attitudes. *Leviticus,* the book of laws, says that after every regular "discharge of blood" a woman is unclean for seven days, and everything she sits or lies on during this time must be considered unclean as well. If a man dares "lie" with her, he will become contaminated. Only after the eighth day can she seek atonement for "her unclean discharge."

The Old Testament rulemakers mistakenly thought, as did the members of other primitive societies, that menstruation was related to uncleanliness, disease, and death, rather than to the nurturing of life. Men have always been in awe of the ability of women to carry a fetus and give birth. Perhaps, men may have reasoned, the body powerful enough to give life is powerful enough to take life.

Because of a woman's known reproductive capabilities, her biology became her destiny. And for many women, it still is. Although it is thousands of years since those Old Testament laws were laid down, some still survive. Orthodox Jewish women and men, for example, are forbidden by the Talmud (a collection of Jewish law and tradition) from having sexual intercourse during a woman's period. Actually, any physical contact at this time is not allowed; a couple's beds may even be separated to ward off sexual temptation. Only after a woman has ritually cleansed herself in the *mikvah,* a special bath, on either the seventh day of her menstrual cycle, or following a miscarriage or giving birth, can she resume sexual relations with her husband.

Most women in modern Western society do not have rules of menstrual behavior spelled out for them. They do, nevertheless, operate under the power of various unwritten strictures. Many women are still brought up to believe that their "time of the month" is one of sickness and weakness.

Mothers, often embarrassed at the thought of explaining menstruation and conception to their young daughters, fall back on euphemism and half-truth. This reticence leads to the proliferation of rumors. "Don't go to the dentist during your menstrual flow. Any fillings put in place will drop right out." "Avoid cold drinks. They are a shock to the system at this sensitive time." "Don't go swimming. It will cause you to hemorrhage."

Sorting fact from fiction can

be very difficult, especially for a confused thirteen-year-old. Despite her pride in her burgeoning womanhood, every young girl must wonder what the onset of menstruation and physical maturation will do to her body. The joys of growing up may be mixed with the fear that her childish, carefree existence is gone forever.

Few women, young or old, call menstruation by its proper name. The expressions "getting my period" or "having the monthlies" are fairly innocent; they simply express the periodic quality of menstrual functioning. But impersonal pronouns or crude slang expressions are more the rule. "Did you get *it* yet?" is the question prepubescent girls most often use to poll their young friends. Another might announce that her "friend" is here. Menstruation is also referred to as the "curse," "having the rag on," or being visited by "Aunt Red" or a "friend from Red Bank." A woman may describe herself as having "fallen off the roof," being "unwell," "sick," or "indisposed." The message is pretty clear.

The Menstrual Role

An outspoken physician named Edgar Berman came to national attention in the late 1960s when he declared that a woman president could be dangerously unstable because she was subject to a "raging hormonal imbalance." The assumption was that, during the time she was menstruating, the female executive just might push the button and blow us all to bits. Despite the warnings of what a menstruating head of state might do to a country, however, nothing so tragic or bizarre has ever happened. (We'll talk about the hormonal question and research being done all over the world in regard to premenstrual syndrome in Chapter Four.)

This is not to say that menstruation hasn't, at least indirectly, played a role in history. A number of fascinating examples follow. But it is important to keep in mind that particularly "masculine" attributes—the ability, or inability, to father an heir, for example—can just as radically affect the future.

In at least two cases, a queen's trouble with menstruation probably changed the course of world events. Elizabeth I was known as the Virgin Queen of England because she never married or had children. Historians have generally assumed that this was because she didn't want to wrestle a man for the power of her throne, but it may be due to a different reason. There is a good chance Elizabeth had a serious fertility problem. Shortly after she assumed the throne in 1558, rumors began circulating that she was sterile. She had infrequent periods and followed a regimen of regular bloodlettings, but these did not correct the problem.

Elizabeth's half sister, Queen Mary I, had no better luck with

Lizzie Borden blamed her period for the blood on her skirt.

menstruation. She suffered from amenorrhea, a serious-sounding condition that simply means a lack of menstrual periods, and tried all the cures of the day. Her inability to have a child caused problems between her and her husband, King Philip of Spain.

If either of these women had had a child, it would have become king or queen of England, and the history of Great Britain might have been very different. But that is not to say that history was therefore affected—adversely or not—solely by gyne-cological factors. There is a good chance both Elizabeth and Mary inherited their barrenness, and syphilis besides, from their father, Henry VIII. Thus, a historian might just as easily argue that it was actually a man who prevented the conception of an heir.

When Joan of Arc was burned at the stake at the age of twenty, she was said never to have menstruated. French historian Jules Michelet claimed that Joan controlled what he called life's "vulgar infirmities" and never suffered the "physical curse of women." Queen Marie Antoinette had the opposite problem. She apparently experienced traumatic menstrual bleeding a few days before she was guillotined in 1793. The morning of her execution, she found her chemise stained red with blood. Rather than suffer the embarrassment—even after death—of having soiled herself, she hid it in the wall behind the stove.

Feminist and anarchist Emma Goldman suffered from irregular and painful periods for most of her life, bleeding when confronted with stress. A physician urged surgery to reduce the pain, but she refused the operation. On the other hand, Virginia Woolf, the British novelist, found the time of her period to be one of great creativity. While she was working on her novel *Orlando*, a story about androgeny, her period came at the same time she broke through an episode of writer's block.

But, possibly the most notorious menstruater was New England ax murderer Lizzie Borden. There is no proof that her period drove her to kill her parents in 1892, but evidence suggests that these famous murders took place during the time of her period. When asked how blood got on her skirt, Lizzie explained that she had "fleas," a Massachusetts euphemism for menstruation. Given the layers of clothing women wore at the time, it was unlikely that a dark spot of menstrual blood had worked its way out from underneath her clothing. But without the technique of blood analysis, this could not be proven; and the discomfort of an all-male jury faced with a woman talking about her period probably obscured the situation and helped lead to her acquittal.

An Absorbing Problem

One reason Lizzie Borden's claim is plausible is that, at the time, control of menstrual flow was awkward and messy. When she menstruated, like the other women of the 1800s, Lizzie Borden probably wore folded rags thick enough to absorb the blood. Once used, they would be rinsed clean, allowed to dry, and stored until her next period.

It was not until 1921 that the first disposable sanitary napkin was introduced. And even then women's magazines did not run ads for them. That would have been considered in poor taste. These magazines did, however, advertise products that could help a woman take care of her homemade menstrual cloths. The *Ladies' Home Journal* and *Good Housekeeping* of the day show print ads for Lysol cleaner, good for "every purpose of personal hygiene." "Amolin: the Personal Deodorant Powder" was touted in the magazines as good for intimate female uses. (Sound familiar? Advertisers are *still* pitching that line to women.)

Tampons were introduced to the American market in the mid-1930s by Tampax, which was incorporated in 1936. At the same time, sanitary napkins were being sold much as they are today. Advertisements promised a woman that her messy secret would not be revealed.

Their major point seemed to be that it was a woman's duty to be in control of her period

What woman hasn't known the sense of personal failure and humiliation when her secret advertises itself on her new white pants or skirt?

During the 1940s, a "sensible" attitude toward menstruation prevailed. There was a war on, and women had to call upon their womanly strengths to help the national war effort. Wartime advertising took females seriously. It called them women, not girls, and emphasized how menstruation didn't have to keep a woman away from her station. Ads in 1943 showed women wearing slacks, getting dressed for work, and carrying lunch pails.

Don't leave a tampon in place more than four hours.

But once women were no longer needed in the work force to win the war, menstrual product advertising reflected this. Women went back to being girls again—beautiful, secretive, and safe. In the "Modess, because" ads that ran in the fifties, impeccably groomed women swathed in yards and yards of diaphanous material posed for pictures looking peaceful and unruffled. The ads were supposedly selling Modess, but I know at least one little girl who thought if she bought Modess when the need arose, she would get to wear glorious dresses, too.

Tampon advertisers took a different tack. Internal protection with tampons had gotten a boost from the wartime emphasis on staying active while menstruating. Tampax advertised that their product was useful for the "woman at home or in the office" as well as for "special users" such as movie stars, bike riders, and swimmers. Tampons were also a boon for women who wore formfitting clothing. Elastic belts with metal hoods held "full-size" napkins more or less in place, but the belts left "telltale lines" and caused pain. The coccyx of many a woman bore a bruise from the pressure of a metal napkin gripper.

For a while, one company tried to sell its product by making it easier to get rid of. Scott Confidets enclosed "neat disposal bags in each box." But most companies focused on other issues. To make napkins more comfortable and probably to capture more of the market, napkin makers started offering the belt-free napkin in the early 1970s. Small strips of adhesive gripped the pad to underpants. These napkins were more comfortable, but the glue often grabbed onto pubic hairs—a new problem.

The women's movement and women's influx into the work force also influenced tampon and napkin makers who now try to sell their products by advertising female professional competence as well. The OB Tampon campaign, advertises that the tampon was designed by a woman gynecologist, reflecting this attitude.

TSS

One of the biggest crises the menstrual products industry had to face involves toxic shock syndrome (TSS), which erupted into a nationwide scare in 1980. Late in 1979, the Center for Disease Control in Atlanta, Georgia, was notified that a half dozen menstruating young women in Wisconsin had been hospitalized with similar symptoms—fever over 102 degrees, dizziness, low blood pressure, rash on the body and soles and palms, nausea and vomiting, diarrhea, and muscle aches. It seemed that women

who used tampons were especially vulnerable to TSS, and some otherwise healthy young women died.

Although the disease has occurred in women using every brand of tampon—as well as a case involving sanitary napkins and another involving sea sponges, a natural product used for absorption—Rely, the newest brand of tampon on the market in 1980, was suspected of making women more susceptible to the disease. More users of Rely got TSS than women who used other brands. Rely's manufacturer, Procter and Gamble, voluntarily withdrew Rely tampons from the market.

Toxic shock syndrome is caused by the absorption of a poison produced by some strains of penicillin-resistant *Staphylococcus aureas*. Even though very few women carry this organism in the vagina or cervix, it may live on the skin of the vulva, the liplike opening to the vagina.

Current hypotheses suggest that tampons don't cause TSS, but inserting them introduces the germ into the vagina. With time, the organism grows in the blood-soaked tampon and is absorbed into the vaginal skin through tiny cuts made in that skin when the tampon was inserted.

Women who still want to use

tampons while they menstruate can cut down on the risk of contracting TSS by following these directions. Wash the vulva completely twice a day when you use tampons. Wash your hands before and after inserting a tampon. Don't leave a tampon in place more than four hours. Alternate tampon use with another method of absorption during a twenty-four-hour period. Wear tampons only when you are flowing heavily. And avoid super-absorbent varieties, which are more likely to cause tiny vaginal lacerations.

It is not thought that TSS will cause the $500-million-a-year feminine personal products industry to seriously suffer. Women who menstruate will continue to choose between napkins and tampons. They will buy *something*. Few, if any, will resort to the homemade, reusable kind of protection.

How much have our attitudes toward menstruation changed?

Product makers would like women to think using what they manufacture will make a menstruating day just like any other. But assurance that the blood will be thoroughly absorbed is not enough. Psychologically, we are just coming out of the Dark Ages as far as menstruation is concerned. Some of the most sophisticated of women still think of themselves as somehow "different" during their menstrual periods, one important reason being that many still experience physical discomfort, including disabling menstrual cramps.

But women in most cases no longer need to be crippled by monthly pain. Research into how the female body works has uncovered the causes of cramps, and we now know how to stop or help ease them.

The major breakthrough for those who suffer, however, was the admission of something these menstruating women already knew: those cramps are real.

CHAPTER TWO

CAN THIS BE NORMAL?

Menstruation is a function of a healthy woman's reproductive system, which occurs twelve or thirteen times annually for some thirty-five years.

In order to understand the menstrual cycle, let's first take a look at the internal organs that make up the female reproductive system.

The reproductive system in a woman is made up of two ovaries, two fallopian tubes, a uterus (the neck of which is called the cervix), and a vagina. These organs are all located in the lower half of a woman's body—her pelvic region—and are connected by a network of ligaments and membranes.

Another important part of the system is the pituitary gland. Located at the base of the brain, it is the body's master gland, manufacturing substances that control the hormone production of many other organs. Acting as a body computer, it cues the beginning and ending of hormone production, and dictates how much of each hormone is made. An area in the midbrain called the hypothalmus "reads" the hormones circulating in the bloodstream and signals the pituitary by means of small molecules—the releasing factors. They are transported directly to the pituitary by a special system of veins. The hypothalmus has connections to many other parts of the brain and is the most sensitive part of the cycling system.

The two ovaries are oval-shaped glands located on either side of the uterus. They are kept from moving around inside the pelvic cavity by a large, leaf-shaped ligament that connects them to the pelvic walls and the uterus. Even though the ovaries can't move very far, they are not rigidly held; they move a lot like testicles do in a man. Actually, the ovaries and the testicles start out at the same place in the developing fetus. If the fetus is female, they stay within the abdominal cavity and develop into ovaries; if it is male, they thicken and drop down through the lower body into the male's scrotal sac. (When the testicles move down and then outside the body, they leave a path that is susceptible to hernias).

The ovaries serve two very important functions. They are the storehouses, ripeners, and re-

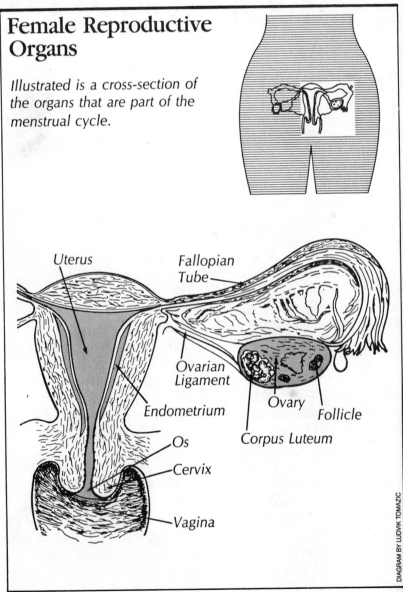

Female Reproductive Organs

Illustrated is a cross-section of the organs that are part of the menstrual cycle.

Uterus

Fallopian Tube

Ovarian Ligament

Endometrium

Ovary

Follicle

Os

Corpus Luteum

Cervix

Vagina

leasers of a woman's eggs, and they are the producers of the female hormones, estrogen and progesterone (more about them later), which run the woman's reproductive system. A female child is born with all the egg-producing follicles she will ever have, and many times more than she will ever need—about a million of them. Many of them have died off by the time she reaches puberty, the age of her first period. Of the approximately ten thousand egg follicles remaining in each ovary, only about four to five hundred will mature over the thirty-five years of her reproductive life.

The ovaries respond to three hormones secreted and controlled by the pituitary gland—the gonadotropins. (The word *gonad* means sex organ or ovary, and *tropic* means effecting or stimulating.) The three are the follicle-stimulating hormone, FSH; the luteinizing hormone, LH; and the luteotrophic hormone, LTH. For the ovary to do its work, a cyclic variation among these three hormones must be achieved and maintained.

The follicle-stimulating hormone's job is to encourage some of the immature egg follicles to grow. It also helps the one egg that does mature fully to push its way out of the ovary. The third function of FSH is to help stimulate the manufacture of the hormone estrogen inside the ovary, and FSH may also help prepare the ovaries to produce progesterone.

LH, the second hormone, governs ovulation. When the mature egg breaks through the ovary wall, the surrounding cells form a yellow body called a corpus luteum which secretes progesterone.

LTH, the third hormone, stimulates the breast glands to produce milk. LTH is commonly called prolactin.

In addition to producing the three ovary-stimulating hormones, the pituitary gland guides the ovaries in their manufacture of estrogen and progesterone, which have a range of influence that extends outside the ovaries.

Estrogen's part in the menstrual cycle is to stimulate the lining of the uterus to grow in preparation for implantation of an egg fertilized by a sperm. The amount of estrogen produced varies with the stages of the menstrual cycle.

Progesterone prepares the lining of the uterus to support life at the beginning of a pregnancy, before the placenta or birth sac is formed. The word *progesterone* comes from the Greek words meaning "favoring birth." Pro-

Menstrual cycles in normal women can range from 17 to 44 days.

duction of progesterone does not start until after the egg is released from the ovary, which is during the second half of a woman's menstrual cycle. In rare cases, women can ovulate more than one egg at a time. Fraternal twins and multiple nonidentical births are the result.

The only way the released egg can get down into the uterus is through the fallopian tubes. The fallopian tubes extend from both sides of the uterus toward the ovaries. These are not rigid runways, but rather flexible cilia, or hair-lined tubes, that provide a passageway for the uterus-bound egg as well as a meeting place for the egg and sperm.

When a fertilized egg does not implant in the uterine lining, progesterone production dramatically declines. This causes the lining of the uterus to break down and come out of the uterus through the os, the opening in the cervix, (the neck of the uterus), which extends into the vagina. This is menstruation.

The Monthlies

Menstruation is the process that enables a new phase of a woman's reproductive cycle to begin, and prepares her body for conception should it occur the next month. The blood in the menses, or menstrual fluid, is due to the breaking of tiny blood vessels in the lining of the uterus, called the endometrium. This blood mixes with the discarded uterine lining and cervical mucus to make up the three to six tablespoons of an average month's flow.

The color and consistency of the menstrual flow can differ. The flow of a healthy woman can vary from bright red to dark, from thin to clotty, and from scanty to floodlike. Women who take birth control pills are more likely to have scant dark red to brown blood, different from their menstrual blood when they are not on oral contraceptives.

The rate of menstrual flow can also vary. Most women report a heavier flow the first day or two and a tapering off after that. Others say their flow is fairly constant during their period.

The word *menstruation* comes from the Latin word for month, *mensis*. Most women mentruate about once a month for approximately thirty-five years. That does not mean they menstruate once in January and one more time for every calendar month of the year, but that about once every twenty-eight days or so the menstrual cycle goes through its stages and starts up again. For many women, the menstrual cycle is monthly, completed in twenty-six to thirty-three days. But cycles in normal women can range from seventeen to forty-four days. A shorter cycle can be a boon to a woman trying to get pregnant. If she is lucky enough to ovulate every cycle, she has more chances in a shorter time to connect with a perm. But most often, a shorter cycle is considered a nuisance.

Too many women who don't conform to the twenty-eight-day average think there is something wrong with them. This is usually not the case. For example, one of my patients complained of periods that were always five days late. She isn't late—she has a thirty-three-day cycle. When a young woman starts to menstruate, generally between the ages of nine and sixteen (in the United States, at approximately 12.3 years of age), her periods can be very irregular. They may come at different intervals; each may last a different number of days, and be of varying volume. After several years, however, her body slowly adjusts to this new function, and her periods become more regular.

In general, young women tend to have more "exotic" cycles than older women. One study found that of the fifteen- to nineteen-year-olds studied, 62 percent had menstrual cycles between twenty-five and thirty-one days long. But with age, the body seems to change. The study shows that of women between thirty-five and thirty-nine years old, 86 percent conformed to the standard cycle.

The Cycle

Let us examine the idealized twenty-eight-day cycle, generally measured by calling the first day of menstrual bleeding Day 1. This cycle is divided by ovulation into two stages.

During the first few days of the cycle, estrogen production starts to increase. This estrogen, produced by the ovaries and transported to the uterus by the vascular system, stimulates the uterine lining—the endometrium—to grow. During the first fourteen days of this hypothetical twenty-eight-day cycle, this lining grows in order to nourish any fertilized egg which may implant there.

At the same time, a number of follicles in the ovary are growing. Some time during the first seven days of the cycle, one follicle takes the lead, developing more rapidly and more fully than the rest. This selected follicle is called the Graafian follicle. It breaks through the ovarian confines at about Day 14. That break is ovulation, the sign that one follicle has won the race. All the other follicles gradually die off.

Ovulation is quick. Some women can feel it. They report a sharp prick in one side of the abdomen, or a longer period of discomfort. Some women have a full day of bleeding at mid-cycle, others just a bit of spotting. Most don't see any discharge, but there is data that suggests that every cycling woman bleeds at ovulation, if only microscopically.

A woman who is ovulating may feel sexier as her matured egg breaks through the ovarian wall. She may also initiate sex more freely at this time. On the other hand, the woman who feels crabby when she ovulates, or who gets abdominal pain or a headache, may want to be left alone.

The woman with a twenty-eight-day cycle usually ovulates at Day 14. Any woman with a longer cycle is likely to ovulate later in her elongated "month." A thirty-five-day menstrual cycle may produce ovulation at Day 21. Someone with a shorter cycle, say twenty-one days, is probably ovulating about Day 7.

With ovulation, the first stage of the menstrual cycle ends. Either the released egg will be fertilized by a male sperm or not. Because there is a delay between the day when a woman ovulates and the time a fertilized egg implants itself in the uterine wall, the uterus continues to prepare itself to nurture the embryo. The second stage of the menstrual cycle in a twenty-eight-day woman runs from Day 15 until Day 28. Until Day 20 or 21, the lining continues to grow. If implantation does not take place, a reversal sets in. The progesterone and estrogen levels decrease, and the endometrial lining breaks down and flows out of the body, returning us to Day 1—the first day of menstruation.

During this post-ovulatory second stage, if fertilization and implantation do occur, the endometrial surface of the uterus becomes more vascular and continues to develop to bring nutrients to the embryo. Some time between Day 24 and Day 26, the levels of estrogen, progesterone, and LH (luteinizing hormone) climb even higher. Mammary glands begin to gear up to produce milk for the newborn baby.

Estrogen can cause the breasts of women who do not get pregnant to swell at this late-cycle time of the month. They may retain fluids in other parts of their bodies as well, fluids that can add as much as five or ten pounds to their weight. This "temporary water weight gain," as one over-the-counter drug advertiser calls it, is technically edema, or swelling. Women with this condition say they feel bloated.

Data suggests that cycling women bleed at ovulation.

For some women, this swelling is more than a minor monthly annoyance. It can be very painful and, in the extreme, distorting. Some women suffer so much that they cannot sleep on their stomachs, and complain that their clothing gets too tight to comfortably wear. I'll talk about how to attack this problem by making changes in diet and exercise or by using medication, both pre-scribed and over-the-counter varieties, in Chapter Four.

Cycle Changes

Although some women experience consistent premenstrual symptoms and menstrual periods during their entire reproductive lives, most women observe that their bodies change with age and with internal and external events.

Young women usually get their first period, or *menarche*, (from the Greek *archē*, "beginning"), at the average age of 12.3, although some don't start menstruating until age sixteen or even later. It is a good idea to have a physician examine any young woman older than sixteen who has not gotten her period; her endocrine and genetic systems as well as sexual organs should be checked. A number of young women who do not menstruate until later than the average age are engaged in some intense physical training program; it appears that they don't have enough fat on their bodies to menstruate. Studies of women ballet dancers show that when body fat drops below 22 percent, menstruation stops. The average twenty-five-year-old has about 26 to 28 percent body fat. Adolescent girls don't need as much fat to menstruate as adults do, but if their fat level dips below 17 percent, this will delay the onset of menstruation and puberty. This fat-level index, along with psychological effects on the cycling center in the brain, explains why young women suffering from anorexia nervosa don't menstruate. These young women are not always engaged in a strenuous physical training program, but usually their fat percentage drops far below the level needed to menstruate.

Environmental stress can often change a woman's cycle.

Women who are very overweight also frequently experience a loss of their periods along with their extreme weight gain. Fat cells may act as reservoirs for estrogen, preventing it from stimulating ovulation and menstruation. And any other physical condition that disturbs the delicate balance of the ovary-stimulating hormones or the production of estrogen or progesterone can also throw the whole process off.

A woman with irregular or nonexistent periods may not be concerned about her cycle until she is either thinking about having a baby or trying to get pregnant and failing. If the reason she is not conceiving turns out to be a failure to ovulate—which in turn is causing her irregular cycle—there are drugs available that can help her to ovulate. These drugs, Clomid and Pergonal, are used to stimulate the ovaries into action.

When it is time for a woman's periods to resume after a pregnancy, she may find that her cycle has totally changed. About a third of the women who suffer painful menstrual cramps find pregnancy has cured them. A full-term pregnancy greatly stretches the uterus and may relieve uncomfortable spasms of that muscle. I'll talk more about this in Chapter Three.

A good many women are susceptible to factors far more elusive than hormonal imbalance. "Environmental stress," for example, can often change a woman's cycle. The trauma of an auto accident can cause a between-periods woman to start flowing on the way to the hospital. The excitement of getting married may bring on an unscheduled period. Worry, illness, even a long airplane ride and a change of climate can make a period suddenly appear or disappear.

What happens when a woman who has had a consistent twenty-eight-day cycle gets a very occasional twenty-four or thirty-five day menstrual period? Unless there are other conditions that cause alarm, her only course of action should be to give thanks that she has always been so regular. Given the intricacies of hormonal balance and internal synchronizing essential for any woman to cycle at all, it is amazing that women are as regular as they are.

But don't ignore signals that something may be wrong with your menstrual cycle and your reproductive system. There *is* a time to go for help. Random intermittent continuous bleeding should be investigated. A single episode of unusual bleeding may be explained by some upheaval, some outside event. But if it recurs report it to your gynecologist.

Menopause

Although the median age in this country when menstrual periods stop—that is, when a woman enters menopause—is 51.4, most women begin to experience greater variation in cycle length, and the amount and duration of flow, some time around the age of forty. The million or so eggs that were created while a woman was in her mother's uterus have by now been reduced to a few thousand. It may be that these remaining eggs are those least responsive to the stimulating effects of the pituitary hormones that cause ovulation, but in any case, the frequency of irregular and different menstruation increases. Estrogen production by the ovaries also gradually stops, although the amount of estrogen circulating in the blood stream remains significant, because a more complex hormone made by the adrenal gland is changed into estrogen in the fatty tissues of the body.

The ten-year period before menopause and the ten years after is referred to by doctors as the climacteric. During these twenty years, women experience a number of symptoms that are related to increased variation in cycle and the end of menstruation: hot flashes, the thinning of the skin of the vulva and vagina, and, for some, an increase in a variety of physical and psychological problems including muscle and joint pain, headaches, insomnia, anxiety, irritability, and mood swings.

Whether these symptoms cause minor annoyance or major

discomfort depends primarily upon individually-inherited genetic tendencies.

Hot flashes are feelings of heat that usually begin in the area of the chest and move up to the head. They are accompanied by perspiration that may range from slight to excessive, which lasts from a few minutes to an hour or so. The severity of the flashes appears to be directly related to the speed with which estrogen production by the ovaries declines. A fast drop in estrogen produces a greater frequency of hot flashes. The more frequent and severe these flashes are, the more likely they will disappear faster.

Women who have their ovaries removed before menopause, for example, experience "surgical menopause," going through a short period when their symptoms are very severe; these symptoms disappear after three to six weeks. Women whose estrogen levels decline gradually, however, may have only a few hot flashes, but they are at greater risk of experiencing irregular bleeding as their estrogen levels wax and wane during the slow decline.

Only about half the women going through menopause experience hot flashes.

In addition to the role estrogen plays in the reproductive cycle of women, it protects the skin of the vulva and the vagina by making it thick, much like the skin on the palm of your hand. As estrogen production decreases, the skin becomes thin, more like the back of the hand. In this thinner state, it is more vulnerable to infection and to trauma than it used to be, although it is still no more suspectible to injury than skin over other parts of the body.

Consistent use of the skin of the vulva and vagina helps preserve and protect it. Women whose sexual activity continues to be regular despite increasing age report that they have few problems after menopause. However, women whose sexual behavior at this time is disrupted by illness, separation, or a decrease in activity for any reason will be more likely to experience difficulties when they resume sex.

A variety of other complaints that accompany estrogen decline, ranging from anxiety, depression, irritability, and fatigue to muscle and joint pain, depend in large measure on two factors: the actual physical health of the woman, and her psychological response to aging.

Some women lose bone mass after menopause. The bones

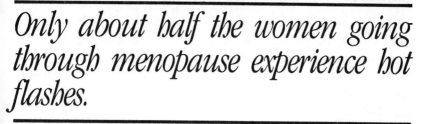

Only about half the women going through menopause experience hot flashes.

supporting the body actually thin, which leads to a shortening of the spine and an increase of fractures—most often of the hip and forearm. This condition is called osteoporosis. For most women, diet and exercise appear to be far more important in preventing osteoporosis than estrogen replacement (taking additional estrogen into the body after the ovaries stop producing it). However, those women who are relatively sedentary or who have well-established osteoporosis appear to benefit from at least a few years of estrogen therapy, which seems to decrease bone mineral loss and to cut down the number of bone fractures.

Estrogen replacement therapy is a medical treatment with both risks and benefits, and it has been hotly debated within the medical community. Among its benefits are control over hot flashes, reversal of any atrophy of the skin of the vagina, and a decrease in urinary symptoms that sometimes occur, such as increased frequency and urgency of urination. The added estrogen also

cuts back the rapid loss of the mineral content of the bones.

The risks of estrogen therapy, however, are significant. Estrogen replacement therapy has definitely been associated with an increase in cancer of the endometrium, the uterine lining. There is one study suggesting that there is a slight increase in breast cancer in women taking estrogen for fifteen years or more, but this is not supported by other surveys. However, estrogen therapy does cause breast cancer in men when given to them as treatment for certain medical conditions.

Estrogen in high doses should not be taken by women with arteriosclerosis, high blood pressure, or diabetes. The birth control pill, which contains both estrogen and progesterone, carries a warning that it should not be given to women over forty because it produces coronary artery disease. Recent studies suggest that estrogen replacement may actually *reduce* coronary artery disease in women whose menopause occurs before the age of forty, but right now, the verdict on the effects of estrogen replacement therapy on women with heart disease is not in.

Finally, estrogen replacement therapy may cause breast tenderness, weight gain, and fluid retention as well as abnormal vaginal bleeding.

Carefully controlled, prospective studies of estrogen replacement therapy are being conducted, but it takes years and large numbers of subjects for conclusive results. Until that data is available, those women who use estrogen replacement therapy should make sure that they get careful and frequent checkups by their doctors. Both these women and their physicians should be alert for any new developments.

CHAPTER THREE

THOSE CRAMPS ARE REAL

Until fairly recently, painful menstruation, or dysmenorrhea (dis-men-oh-ree-uh) as it is known in the medical world, was generally thought to be due to some unexplained psychologcal condition. The pain, it was hypothesized, could be cured by mind over menstruation. In fact, a huckster with a course in the Power of Positive Periods could have done well, and in some places still could.

Although the news has not reached everyone, those cramps are real. As early as the 1930s medical researchers compared menstrual cramps to angina, the muscle cramps that cause men and women terrible chest pain. Apparently, angina is physiologically similar to the uterine muscle cramps of primary dysmenorrhea, a condition that shows up early in a woman's reproductive life, shortly after she begins to menstruate. (Secondary dysmenorrhea, which occurs later in the reproductive years, may be due to something abnormal, such as fibroids or endometriosis. We discuss this condition later in this chapter, on page 35.) But this research seems to have been hidden for decades; until recently, women were told that their cramps were probably in their heads, representing some internal conflict with their femininity.

But, like the real pain of angina, menstrual cramps are real, too. They just occur in a different organ.

Unfortunately, there are some health professionals who are not up-to-date with the advances in research, drug development, exercise, and nutritional guidance that can bring women monthly relief. Instead, they may only prescribe traditional painkillers and dole out condescension to those patients who experience monthly discomfort. It may be because so little help has been available over the years that a recent National Health Examination study reports that few adolescent women see their doctors even for severe menstrual pain. They feel they have to grimace and bear it.

But there is help available. Many family physicians, pediatricians, and gynecologists, as well as college health personnel, and company nurses and doctors, know the extent of the problem of painful periods and are aware of the new methods of relieving the discomfort.

The menstruating years of a woman's life, ranging from the onset of menarche—her first period—to menopause, some thirty-five years later, are ones of study and work. This time is

---

Being unable to prevent the pain can make a woman feel powerless.

---

too important to be disrupted twelve times annually by a physical condition that can be avoided.

How an adolescent young woman reacts to her early menstruation can color her whole life. In the extreme, a girl with pain-

ful periods may in some ways refuse to grow up. Who wants to leave behind a childhood that has to look carefree by comparison and embrace a painful womanhood? Some women retreat, avoiding social contacts. Others are psychologically damaged, by both the memory of those painful cramps and the fact that they will almost certainly return with a flip of the calendar.

A good many women put up with the dread and the pain, hoping for relief as they get older. About a third of the women who suffer from primary dysmenorrhea do get relief after they have children. Roughly another third of the women find their cramps stay the same. But for an unlucky 10 percent or so, cramps get worse.

Several studies show that women who have painful periods sometimes turn the stress of dealing with that condition inward. Anxiety and menstruation that is even more painful can result. Being "sick" monthly and being unable to prevent the pain can make a woman feel powerless, without a sense of self-determination or autonomy. This can affect her entire personality.

These debilitating effects start early. It is estimated that at least 10 percent of teen-age girls are absent from school every month because of menstrual pain. That, according to observers in both the United States and the Scandinavian countries, makes painful menstruation the number one reason why young women miss class.

Because of these absences or because their concentration in class is disturbed by discomfort, women with dysmenorrhea, at least in one study, have shown lower grades and more school adjustment problems than women without menstrual pain.

These Things Called Cramps

Menstrual cramps are caused by contractions of the uterus, which is a muscle. Every woman has a distinct pattern of uterine activity, as individual as her fingerprint. Normal hormonal activity causes the uterus to contract and relax all month long, but usually the contractions are frequent and short in duration. At the time of menstruation, the uterus undergoes stronger, more frequent contractions.

Both before a woman's monthly flow begins and during the first few days of her period, hormone–like substances called prostaglandins are at higher levels in her body.

The pioneering work done on the role of prostaglandins in the menstrual cycle was carried out during the late 1950s and early 1960s by Dr. Vernon Pickles at England's Sheffield University. He called prostaglandins "menstrual stimulants," and identified them in menstrual flow.

Since synthetic prostaglandins are effective in starting a woman's labor and in bringing on second trimester abortions (both of which involve uterine contractions), the natural prostaglandins produced by a woman's body are thought to contract the uterine muscle at the time of menstruation. It also turns out, Dr. Pickles observed in 1965, that some women who report painful periods actually have more of these prostaglandins in their bodies than women who don't.

Women who suffer from dysmenorrhea have uterine contractions that are particularly violent. In addition, there is less time between each contraction—which means the uterus is less often relaxed and pain-free. One condition that accompanies this high uterine activity level is that local blood circulation is often nearly cut off from the uterus. This doesn't affect the menstrual flow, but the lack of oxygenated blood makes the nerve endings even more sensitive, causing the contractions to feel worse.

One of the reasons we know so much about how the uterus flexes at the time of menstruation is because women have allowed themselves to be observed. The earliest successful experiment that measured the activity of a nonpregnant uterus was conducted by a Finnish researcher named Heinricius, in 1889, using a thin rubber bag. For more than fifty years, uterine action was charted by using different balloon techniques. In the 1930s, C. Moir inserted a small rubber balloon into the uteri of women with severe dysmenorrhea. He also gave the women rubber bags to hold in their hands. The women were instructed to squeeze the bag as each cramp increased in intensity. Simultaneously, he recorded how much pressure was exerted on the balloon inside the uterus. He found that the worst pain occurred from just after the peak of the uterine contraction until the uterus had relaxed completely.

Writing in the *Journal of the American Medical Association* in 1947, a research team headed by R. A. Woodbury reported on their study of women who suffered from painful menstruation and women who didn't. Pain-free women enjoyed both reasonable periods of relaxation of the uterus between contractions and a constant flow of blood to the uterus; suffering women showed uteri with uneven patterns of contraction and relaxation. Their conclusion: "The pain of dysmenorrhea is not just psychic in such patients."

Medical researchers have given up their balloons; microtransducers—tiny pressure indicators—are now being placed in women to record more details of the contraction pattern of the nonpregnant uterus. These sophisticated instruments document even more clearly that cramps are physical, not figments of an injured psyche.

Painful Menstruation

Painful menstruation is divided into two different categories by the medical community. The first is fittingly called primary dysmenorrhea, and begins shortly after a young woman starts to menstruate.

Primary dysmenorrhea usually does not show up with a young girl's first period. Most young women who suffer from menstrual pain start having discomfort from six months to two years after they start to menstruate. Many studies point out that painful menstruation goes hand in hand with ovulation. Early cycles may not release ripe eggs, but as a young woman matures, she generates more estrogen and releases mature ova from her ovaries. Unfortunately, along with her hair and eye color, this young woman may well have inherited a genetic predisposition to period pain.

Primary dysmenorrhea is the presence of menstrual pain when nothing is wrong with a woman's menstrual system; secondary dysmenorrhea is caused by something that *has* gone wrong. Secondary dysmenorrhea is a condition that develops later in life, because of disease or other complications. One of the conditions that causes the pain of secondary dysmenorrhea is endometriosis, in which uterine lining appears in the abdominal cavity. The cause of endometriosis is not known, but endometriosis can scar the fallopian tubes, or cause the pelvic organs to stick to each other, and become fixed in the abdominal cavity.

Fibroids and occasionally uterine polyps can also cause pain. And wearing an intrauterine birth control device (IUD) may cause discomfort both at the time of menstruation and between periods.

Whereas the treatment for primary dysmenorrhea may be drugs, exercise, diet change, or even pregnancy, the treatment for the secondary condition may be, of necessity, surgery or drug therapy.

What Cramps Feel Like

We've talked about what causes cramps, but what do they feel like? What does dysmenorrhea do to a body? Women report any number of different sensations, from a dull, throbbing, full-feeling pain across the abdomen under the navel to intense, piercing pain in the same area. The sensation can extend around to the back, with pain radiating up and down the spinal column, and even down one or both legs. The entire perineum, the tissues of the genitals, may feel raw and tender.

Women also complain of having to urinate frequently, and of diarrhea, nausea, and sometimes vomiting. The worst of the symptoms subside after the first day or two.

Painful menstruation and labor pains are both caused by prostaglandins, and many women who suffer terribly every month are told their cramps are like mild labor pains. That comparison makes some women quake with fear. How will they be able to bear the pain of childbirth which they suspect is several times worse than their severe monthly cramps?

Some of these women are in for a pleasant surprise, especially those of them who take prepared childbirth classes and learn relaxation and breathing techniques. These women expect to have some discomfort when they labor to give birth to their children, so they prepare for it; they are therefore more capable of dealing with it. Some expectant women who've suffered from terrible cramps have been delighted to discover that labor wasn't worse, or in some cases labor wasn't as bad, as their monthly pain.

Relief From Menstrual Pain

A woman who suffers from crippling monthly menstrual pain need not resign herself to one or two days a month in bed. She doesn't have to dream of staying pregnant to be free of uterine cramps. She doesn't have to resort to a hysterectomy, as some women have, to get rid of the muscle that is causing her monthly anguish.

There is help available that allows a woman suffering from dysmenorrhea to remain whole and free of pain. The knowledge of how a woman's body works, combined with medical savvy, can equal relief for many.

Over-the-counter medications. The most recent breakthroughs in pharmaceutical aid for menstrual discomfort have been in prescription drugs, but nonprescription remedies remain helpful for many. If you suffer from mild cramps or occasional cramps, products available on drugstore shelves may offer all the help you need.

There are two categories of drugs that are recommended for menstrual distress. First are pain relievers; second are the diuretics, usually taken to release the fluid buildup some women experience before their periods.

Two analgesics, or painkillers, available over the counter are aspirin and acetaminophen. The latter is the active ingredient in nonaspirin pain relievers such as Tylenol; you'll also find it in specific menstrual cramp medications such as Pamprin and Femcaps.

Aspirin is an anti-inflammatory drug that reduces fever and inflammation. It also reduces the amount of prostaglandins pro-

Be aware that almost all drugs have side effects.

duced, thereby cutting down the prostaglandin-encouraged contraction of the uterus and lessening discomfort.

Aspirin also works as an anticoagulant. In other words, it may help keep menstrual blood clots from forming. These clots can cause discomfort when they pass through the os, the opening in the cervix.

Several other nonprescription medications claim to relieve pain by offering ingredients that will relax the pelvic and uterine muscles, thereby decreasing contractions. Cinnamedrine hydrochloride, for example, is an ingredient found in the commercial product Midol. Even though there is no concrete scientific proof that cinnamedrine cuts down on contractions, the Midol manufacturers say their customers feel it does provide relief. Another active agent, atrophine sulfate, is a muscle relaxant used in the commercial product Femcaps.

A number of over-the-counter preparations claim to lessen water retention, but whether these diuretics are effective is questionable. They contain either ammonium chloride or pamabrom. If you choose to try one of the many commercial products containing ammonium chloride (Aqua-Ban or Pre-Mens Forte are two), you will notice they don't contain aspirin. Ammonium chloride is less effective in the presence of aspirin. Therefore, if you need a pain reliever as well as a diuretic, choose one that contains acetaminophen.

Be aware that almost all drugs have side effects, even those sold over the counter. Aspirin, as helpful as it can be for pain, can irritate the stomach. The muscle relaxant atrophine sulfate has been known to cause blurry vision and agitation. Some of the stronger prescription drugs can be habit-forming or make you feel sleepy and less alert.

Prescription drugs. The most common and least expensive painkiller available by prescription is codeine usually prescribed in combination with aspirin or acetaminophen which enhance its effectiveness. It can begin to work a quarter to a half hour after it is taken and may be effective for about four hours.

Antiprostaglandins are a breakthrough treatment for cramps.

The side effects of codeine are not generally serious, but you may develop an allergic skin reaction, an upset stomach, or feel slightly drunk. Don't take codeine at the same time you are taking a diuretic. The combination can make your blood pressure drop dangerously.

The drug oxycodone (present in Percocet-5, Percodan, and Percodan-Demi) takes effect within about an hour and stays active for four to five hours. This drug is a narcotic to which you can become addicted. Withdrawal symptoms are severe. However, if this painkiller is taken once in a while, under careful medical supervision, the side effects are seldom serious. They may include itchy skin, nausea and vomiting, and dizziness.

Pentazocine (Talwin) can remain effective for three or more hours, and begins to work about a quarter to a half hour after taking it, but even if it is used according to doctor's orders, possible side effects can be severe. These include hallucinations and strange behavior, difficulty in urinating, and a slowing down of the production of blood cells. Other possible reactions are hives, swelling and other skin reactions, flushing and sweating, dizziness, headache, and upset stomach.

A last prescription painkiller is propoxyphene (Darvon, Apap, Wygesic, and others). This drug takes an hour or sometimes longer to take effect. There is some question as to how helpful it is. It has never been proven more effective than aspirin, except when it is combined with aspirin or with acetaminophen. Possible side effects from the drug are dizziness, nausea and vomiting, headache, skin rashes, and mild changes in behavior. It may also cause insomnia.

Birth control pills for cramps.
Some women who suffer menstrual cramps and want protection from an unwanted pregnancy take oral contraceptives to ease their pain.

There are good reasons why physicians prescribe birth control pills for painful periods. Besides offering contraception, the chemicals in the pill suppress the production of uterine lining, which reduces monthly menstrual fluid. Also, low levels of prostaglandins are produced during pill-taking cycles, when there is no ovulation.

But not everyone should use the birth control pill to relieve painful menstruation. The pill is, after all, a combination of synthetic hormones that suppress ovulation. The triggering mechanism in the mid brain is inhibited so no egg is released, and no uterine lining thickened to nurture the fertilized egg.

But fooling yourself is not necessarily helping yourself. Women who have taken the birth control pill to regulate erratic menstrual cycles are not being cured of whatever condition may exist that is making them irregular; they are only masking their symptoms. A pill-taker bleeds after she stops taking the pill each month as a physical reaction to the withdrawal of the hormone. Any woman who was not menstruating before she took the pill may therefore seem to menstruate when she is on the pill, but when she finally stops the medication and tries to get pregnant, she may find her erratic periods have resumed. For example, if she was not ovulating

before she took the pill, she will not automatically ovulate when she stops.

Other than masking conditions a woman may want corrected, there are other contraindications for the use of birth control pills for menstrual problems. One of these is age. The pill is not recommended for any woman over thirty-five. Smokers should not take them, nor should women given to migraine headaches or high blood pressure. Anyone who gets dizzy or depressed while on the pill should be taken off it.

Women who take oral contraceptives should be monitored carefully for an initial three- or four-month period. If a woman responds well to the treatment and chooses to stay with it, she should be checked periodically by her physician.

Antiprostaglandins

The most dramatic breakthrough in the treatment of dysmenorrhea has been the development and use of antiprostaglandins, or prostaglandin inhibitors. From our earlier discussion of prostaglandins, you will remember that they are the substances, produced and distributed through the body, that cause contractions of the uterus.

As English researcher Dr. Vernon Pickles noticed, there seem to be more prostaglandins in the menstrual flow of women who suffer from painful periods than in the flow of women who do not.

In 1972, Pickles suggested that maybe an anti-inflammatory drug would cut down prostaglandin production and with it, pain. Aspirin, as we pointed out, is an anti-inflammatory that decreases the prostaglandin level. Pickles suggested that a drug prescribed for relief of arthritis pain in England in 1972 be tried. That anti-inflammatory drug, indomethacin, had never before been promoted as a treatment for menstrual cramps.

Then, in 1974, a quartet of Israeli doctors published a paper in the *Journal of Obstetrics and Gynecology* concerning an experiment they had run treating primary dysmenorrhea. Drs. A. Schwartz, U. Zor, H. E. Lindner, and S. Naor decided to try a nonsteroid, anti-inflammatory drug from the fenamate family, flufenamic acid, on sixteen women with painful cramps. They chose a fenamate (in this case Flunalgan, which is manufactured in Israel) because that family of drugs is known to stop prostaglandin production and to block the action of them on smooth, involuntary muscle, in this case the uterus.

In the thirty-one cases treated, women reported relief while they took the drug and a return of pain when they stopped medication. The physicians also treated the same group of patients with inactive placebos and with tranquilizers, but the women did not get relief from the suggestion of help; they were helped by the action of the drug.

Since the middle of the 1970s, more physicians and patients have become aware of the synthetic prostaglandin inhibitors and what they can do. Research is not complete on any long-term use of the drugs, but the antiprostaglandins have several properties in their favor. They are not steroids. They are not synthetic substances that fool the body into a simulated condition, as do birth control pills. They are not taken three weeks out of every four, as are oral contraceptives, which hold the body in a state of false pregnancy, precluding the need for a mature egg or uterine lining.

Prostaglandin inhibitors are different. They are taken as needed for pain, often as seldom as one day a month. They decrease the production of prostaglandins and signal the uterus to relax. This means the men-

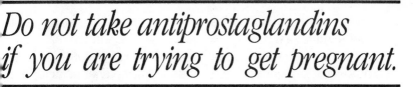

Do not take antiprostaglandins if you are trying to get pregnant.

struating woman can relax, too.

Most menstrual pain lasts somewhere between two and seventy-two hours. For some women, the pain begins before the flow does; for other, it follows. To gain the most relief and be free of even the slightest twinges, a woman can take antiprostaglandins a few days before her period begins. This will both keep the production of prostaglandins down and prevent them from circulating. However, a woman who takes antiprostaglandins in this preventive manner should be aware of certain risks.

The antiprostaglandins have not been in use long enough to know what harm, if any, they do to a fetus. If you are trying to get pregnant or if you think you might be pregnant, taking the prostaglandins before your period starts may damage the embryo. Since some pregnant women feel twinges during the first few months at the time they would usually menstruate, don't think that a slight cramping is proof you are not pregnant. Even if it means tolerating a few hours of discomfort, it is safer to let actual menstrual blood signal the time to take any drug.

Before committing yourself to long-term medication, you and your doctor should conduct a six-month trial. During that time, the specific drug or dosage may be changed, to find what works best for you. Even if your symptoms indicate you have painful periods because of your prostaglandin level, you may not respond to the antiprostaglandins. A woman with secondary dysmenorrhea, for example—endometriosis, fibroids, or ovarian cysts—may find antiprostaglandins offer little or no relief.

There are some women who are neither helped by the antiprostaglandins nor have anything physically wrong with them. In fact, the reason for their cramps may prove to be psychological. But assuming cramps are psychologically caused should be a last, not first, resort.

Here are some of the prostaglandin inhibitors in use:

Fenoprofen (NALFON) is a painkiller that blocks nerve endings; it is also an anti-inflammatory agent.

Ibuprofen (MOTRIN) provides

relief from moderate pain and is an anti-inflammatory.

Indomethacin (INDOCIN) is not yet approved by the Food and Drug Administration as a pain-killer. It is used to treat arthritis, and studies show it relieves menstrual pain.

Mefenamic acid (PONSTEL— PONSTAN IN ENGLAND AND CANADA) is a painkiller related to the flufenamic acid described in the 1974 Israeli report. It is also an anti-inflammatory.

Naproxen (NAPROSYN) and *naproxen sodium* (ANAPROX) are prostaglandin inhibitors. Don't combine these with aspirin.

With any drug, there is always the possibility of side effects—another reason why you and your physician should monitor your reactions to medication and be aware of any allergies you may have.

Many of these drugs can irritate the stomach lining, but this side effect is generally seen in people who take them continuously for other conditions, such as arthritis. Women who take the drugs a few days a month for menstrual cramps almost never develop stomach irritation.

Naproxen, indomethacin, and fenoprofen may inhibit a woman's ability to think clearly or to concentrate. The drugs naproxen and ibuprofen may make the skin erupt. Ibuprofen, indomethacin, mefenamic acid, and zomepirac may interfere with the urinary tract. Ibuprofen, indomethacin, and naproxen can cause depression and bloating.

Since you can get your period while you are nursing, be very careful what drugs you take to relieve cramping at that time. Acetaminophen, aspirin, indomethacin, and naproxen pass through you into your baby's milk.

Some women complain of gastrointestinal upsets that accompany painful menstruation; Those drug's digestive complications may be minimized by taking them with a glass of water or with milk, or with food.

And don't forget that drugs may not be the only answer. Heating pads do help, as does a massage. Orgasm has been known to relieve pelvic congestion and pain. And the kind of exercises that help you stretch out and help you learn to relax muscles, when performed both at the time of menstruation and throughout the month, can also bring relief. I've provided dozens of useful exercises in Chapter Five to help you.

CHAPTER FOUR

PREMENSTRUAL SYNDROME

Not many women are taken by surprise when their monthly menstrual flow begins. They do not have to check the last circle on the calendar to add pads or tampons to their shopping list. Many suffer before the fact from an array of symptoms that are grouped under the heading of premenstrual syndrome (PMS).

Premenstrual symptoms usually appear late in the cycle and at the same point every month. What are the symptoms of PMS and why do they occur?

Water retention. Instead of passing through the system, water is retained in the tissues. It may collect in the ankles, legs, fingers, abdomen, and breasts. Intestinal motility decreases, making you feel constipated, bloated, and heavy.

Fluids stay in a woman's body at this time of the month because of the hormone shift, which causes a change in the potassium-sodium balance. This makes some women retain fluids until

these hormones shift once again, when menstruation occurs and the fluids pass out of the body. Some women gain from four to seven pounds each month before they menstruate. Occasionally, a woman will gain as much as an additional fourteen pounds, and may need to own a second, large-size wardrobe for those days.

Tender breasts. Premenstrual syndrome sufferers frequently say their breasts swell and are sore. Excess water held in the breast tissues can make them tender, even painful, to the touch. Also, the raised estrogen level just before menstruation increases blood flow through the skin and causes pain in some women.

Food cravings. The hormone shift in the second half of the menstrual cycle makes some women crave all sorts of sweet, high-carbohydrate foods such as chocolate, ice cream, and cake. During the first half of the cycle, a woman's blood sugar level can drop considerably lower before she feels hungry or weak or experiences any other symptom indicating that her blood sugar needs replenishing; but during the second half of the cycle, after she ovulates, her blood sugar does not have to drop as much before she needs more food for fuel. Falling down on a diet at this time of the month may be due to a physical need to raise the blood sugar level, not a lack of moral fiber.

Headache. Women complain of two kinds of premenstrual headaches. The first, migraines, are caused by blood vessels in the head expanding and contracting in response to stress alone or stress combined with hormone changes. The second, an ache felt around the temples, is caused by increased muscle tension in the neck and jaw.

Some women feel a little queasy when they have even a slight headache, and these women don't eat. This compounds the low blood sugar problem, and makes them feel even worse.

Clumsiness. One of the symptoms some women often overlook is premenstrual clumsiness. Awkwardness at this time of the month is not totally understood, although it could be due to ten-

sion. Women report that right before their periods, they are more likely to burn themselves at the stove, cut themselves with kitchen knives, and bump into things. G. J. Erdelyi studied female athletes and found some of them performed most poorly during the few days before they got their periods and the first two days of menstruation.

Tension, anxiety, and irritability. The physical symptoms of premenstrual tension are sometimes easier to deal with than the psychological ones because they are more tangible. Psychological symptoms make many women feel like they are possessed.

Women report being jumpy, out of sorts, and on such a short fuse that the slightest thing can cause blowups with family and colleagues.

Depression, too, is a common premenstrual complaint. Women may feel a little teary and blue for a day or two, or face several days of serious depression.

Change in energy levels. A day or two before a period is due is the time some women literally run out of steam. They complain they can't get moving and are tempted to go back to bed as soon as they get up. Any drop

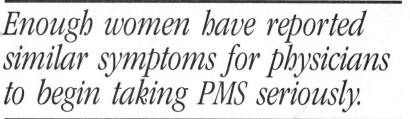

Enough women have reported similar symptoms for physicians to begin taking PMS seriously.

in blood sugar level at this time can make a woman feel even more tired. And a gross imbalance in her sodium-potassium levels can also make her feel worn out.

More rare are the women who say they go into overdrive right before they menstruate. Energy seems to flood into them, giving them the ability to take on projects that would tax several workers. After this gush of energy, however, they say they almost literally collapse, totally drained.

PMS Sufferers

It is estimated that about 30 percent of menstruating women suffer from some degree of premenstrual syndrome. That's some nine to twelve million women in the United States alone. When a study was made of premenstrual syndrome in other parts of the world, Japanese women reported fewer premenstrual symptoms than Turkish, Nigerian, and American women. Headache was the most fre-

quent complaint among Indians, Nigerians, and black Americans.

In 1931 premenstrual syndrome was called premenstrual tension, because women complained of irritability, anxiety, and nervous tension before they menstruated every month.

Even though a good many health professionals and lay people admitted the syndrome existed, most were willing to write it off as psychological. *She's anticipating period pain. She has a hostile, dependent relationship with her mother. She experiences a debilitating envy of men. She's reacting to the stress-filled world she lives in.* But this is not the case. Enough women have reported similar symptoms for physicians to begin taking PMS seriously. It does exist, and it is probably caused by both physical and psychological factors. Unfortunately, researchers have not yet been able to pin it down. PMS is not unlike a vampire. We may hold a scientific mirror up to it, but we haven't yet seen its reflection.

In 1968, Stanford University's Rudolph H. Moos conducted a survey to determine who suffered from symptoms of premenstrual syndrome and when. The results were later published in *Comprehensive Psychiatry*. Moos used both male and female college students, and he didn't tell his subjects the goal of the study. His attempt to prove PMS exists was not totally successful. Each person was asked to record his or her feelings and symptoms for thirty days. On the whole, both male and female students reported the same symptoms and degree of suffering. More women than men did mention sharp and dull aching cramps, pain, and bloating, and women who were due to get their periods soon rated themselves as experiencing more pain, water retention, and abnormal eating habits. But the ideal study on premenstrual syndrome has yet to be done.

Women who suspect they do suffer from premenstrual syndrome to some degree, or who experience other problems they think are unrelated to their menstrual cycle, may learn more about themselves by charting their cycles each day for several months.

Make Day 1 the first day you menstruate. Put down *M* for menstruating, and *C* if and when you have cramps. Indicate your other symptoms day by day: headache, mild or severe; tension; bloating; sore breasts; food cravings.

Observe from month to month if there is a pattern to your complaints, and if there is, it should help you to better understand how you will feel during the various phases of your cycle. You may also discover a pattern that is unrelated to your period. In one case, a woman got headaches every Thursday for several months; then the headaches started skipping Thursdays and occurring every other Tuesday. A change in her menstrual cycle? At first she thought so, but after really thinking it through, she realized there was another cause. During the busy season at work, she had stayed late every Thursday to help her boss. She used to hold off eating dinner until very late, and while they worked he smoked cigars some would call aromatic. She called them stinky. When the busy season slackened and she only worked overtime every other Tuesday, her headaches diminished. There was no menstrual trouble here. The problem was low blood sugar, hunger, and lack of good ventilation.

Causes of PMS

Why do some women suffer from PMS? Some researchers, such as British physician Katherina Dalton, who has been studying and treating PMS for more than thirty years, and Dr. Michael G. Brush and Professor R. W. Taylor of the St. Thomas' Hospital in London, believe that PMS is a result of imbalanced progesterone and estrogen levels in the body. This has never been scientifically substantiated, although one thing does appear clear. PMS is related to the rise and fall of hormones in a woman's body, or, in other words, the ebb and flow of the menstrual cycle. Women on the pill, which produces a more constant level of hormones, rarely suffer from PMS symptoms. Women who are pregnant, a state when the body is a veritable progesterone factory designed to nourish the placenta, don't have PMS either. Ironically, however, a good many women develop premenstrual syndrome for the first time after those nine "carefree" months of pregnancy. No one knows exactly why.

Some students of human history believe women were not meant to menstruate, as most do today, uninterrupted for years. With the reliable birth control methods available today, women are free of pregnancy or nursing for most of their menstruating lives. Since women now menstruate more often than nature intended them to, these historians theorize, premenstrual syndrome is more common.

Progesterone Treatment

Prompted both by her own premenstrual migraines and cases that came her way in 1948, Dr. Katherina Dalton decided that she wanted to help solve the monthly problem that she saw wrecking lives. In 1953 she published the first British medical paper on the subject of premenstrual syndrome, in which she claimed that women are extremely unstable and bizarre in their behavior the four days before their periods begin and the first four days of their cycles. She called this eight-day period the paramenstrum. During the paramenstrum, according to Dr. Dalton, women are more likely to have accidents, attempt to kill themselves, or commit crimes against others. Dalton noted that at four of London's teaching hospitals, 52 percent of the women who were admitted due to accidents were in their paramenstrum.

In Great Britain progesterone is still regularly prescribed for PMS.

A major criticism of these data is that they are incomplete. Granted these women were "paramenstrual," but what was the relationship of this period to their regular cycling schedule. Were they early or on time? What about the periods of the other 48 percent—were they on time or late? It has been suggested by Dr. Mary Parlee, director of the Center for the Study of Women and Sex Roles, City University of New York, Graduate Center, that stress shifts the onset of menstruation away from the norm and, indeed, her analysis of some of Dalton's own data involving British schoolgirls taking university entrance exams supports this theory.

Dr. Dalton believes that this unstable behavior is caused by a dramatic drop in the progesterone level in the body and has treated hundreds of women suffering from PMS with progesterone, saying it alleviates their symptoms.

However, the Dalton theory has never been tested in a carefully controlled, double-blind study to determine its validity. A double-blind study is one in which neither subjects nor researchers know who is being medicated and who is taking a placebo until all the information is gathered and evaluated.

Other researchers who have tried to duplicate Dalton's work have not been able to come up with the same results. Dr. Gwyneth Sampson performed a double-blind study, using some thirty-nine patients in Sheffield, England, doling out to some of the women the exact amount of progesterone Dalton used and giving a placebo to the rest. Sampson found no difference between the two.

Dr. Dalton and others in Great Britain, however, still regularly prescribe progesterone for PMS sufferers. The natural progesterone they use, derived from yams, is taken in vaginal or rectal suppositories. Some women with more virulent symptoms are given progesterone injections. Dalton says the progesterone treatments are essential to correct hormonal systems that are so unbalanced they make monsters of their owners. In fact, progesterone treatments have been accepted so completely in Great

Britain that in three different murder trials there, women have been "sentenced" to take progesterone. In all three cases—one of a woman who killed her baby, another of a woman who ran over her lover with a car, and a third in which a woman prisoner killed another woman inmate—the defense was that they were premenstrual. In addition, the first two had exacerbated their hormonal crisis by not eating for nine hours before their crimes. Instead of going to jail, two of these women are only going to the pharmacist. They were sentenced to progesterone therapy. (The third, already in prison, remained there, but is also taking progesterone.)

Some doctors and women welcome the decisions in these murder cases, hoping they will raise the investigation of PMS to a higher priority. Other women are made very uneasy by them. The issue of a PMS defense stirs up memories of Dr. Edgar Berman, that physician who warned that women couldn't function as rational executives because of monthly "raging hormonal imbalances" (see page 13). All this puts women in a very defensive position. The British cases and the Berman thesis are based on the belief that PMS makes at least some women not just a little teary-eyed or jumpy, but violent, irrational, and murderous. Yet with all this discussion of PMS, women still commit only 10 percent of all violent crimes.

The first PMS defense in a United States criminal trial has recently been mounted in New York, but progesterone therapy has been here for a while. In 1980, the first PMS clinic opened in Reading, Massachusetts, a suburb of Boston. Clinic director Dr. Ronald Norris is a disciple of Dr. Katherina Dalton. He and his staff both diagnose and treat women who come to them for relief from PMS symptoms. Patients have come from all over the county.

Norris believes in Dalton's natural progesterone therapy and currently imports the medication from Great Britain for his patients. It has not been approved by the United States Food and Drug Administration and so is unavailable in America. Dr. Norris is lobbying the FDA and conducting an FDA-approved study in an attempt to gain FDA approval.

What to Do About PMS

Although there are claims from Britain that natural progesterone therapy carries no risks, there are other PMS aids to try before resorting to progesterone.

First, a woman should exercise. A series of conditioning and problem-solving exercises appears in Chapter Five. If fluids are being retained in the tissues, exercise will help move them back into the bloodstream. Exercise also aids the whole vascular system by feeding oxygenated blood to the entire body. And exercise increases the production of those brain chemicals that promote a feeling of well-being.

A woman should also eat wisely. During the second half of the cycle, when your blood sugar level is more vulnerable, make sure your diet is rich in foods that will sustain your blood sugar level. Proteins and complex carbohydrates will stay with you longer than candies and ice cream, which provide a sugar rush that dissipates quickly. If you want something that tastes sweet, put some honey in your tea, and have a piece of cheese with it. Sometimes, spreading out your daily caloric intake over six meals instead of three will prevent headaches, shakiness, and irritability.

Some people advise PMS sufferers to cut out caffeine and cut down drastically on their fluid intake during the second half of the cycle. Others say caffeine makes no difference to premenstrual sufferers. See what works best for you. Record what you eat and drink, and when. Observe if a change in caffeine or

Exercise can often promote a feeling of well-being.

fluid intake alters your symptoms in any way.

Limiting salt intake in the second half of the cycle can help cut down fluid retention. Some women, instead of eliminating salt, increase potassium-rich foods such as dark green leafy vegetables and dark breads, which help them to pass fluid out of their bodies.

Various medications are also prescribed to deal with PMS. **Diuretics.** The progesterone level in a woman's body rises right before her period, encouraging her body tissues to take in and retain water. Fluids that normally pass through the body are, in effect, dammed up until the low begins. When the progesterone level drops again, the fluid is passed through the body and out. But while the problem exists, diuretics are often prescribed. Diuretics, commonly known as "water pills," increase urination.

Two popular diuretics are furosemide (Lasix) and the members of the thiazide family. Furosemide is the more powerful of the two. It takes effect inside of an hour and stays effective for as long as eight hours. This diuretic may be accompanied by nausea and vomiting, diarrhea, and skin rashes, as well as dizziness and blurred vision. Under its brand name, Lasix, it is very popular in the United States, and was the eighth most frequently prescribed drug in the early 1970s. Despite its popularity, however, I think it should not be taken for PMS.

Effective and far more safe are the thiazides, including bendroflumethiazide (Nasturetin), chlorothiazide (Diuril), and hydrochlorothiazide (Esidrix, Hydrodiuril). This family of drugs takes effect after about two hours and can last as long as twelve hours. Possible side effects include dizziness and lightheadedness, loss of appetite, hives, and skin rashes, as well as an allergic reaction to sunlight.

Another helpful diuretic for many women with premenstrual fluid retention is triamterene (Dyrenium). This drug works directly on the kidneys to release salt and water. It does not lower blood pressure, nor does it cause a loss of potassium, both of which are effects of the thiazides and furosemide.

There are a number of precautions to take before and while using diuretics. The powerful ones can work too well, pumping out fluid in great volume and possibly upsetting the electrolyte (water and salt) balance that makes our bodies run. Whenever the potassium level in a woman's body drops too low, she can get weak and develop muscle aches and cramps as well as spasms. Extreme depletion can lead to death. While you are taking a diuretic, check with your doctor immediately if you ever feel excessively thirsty, if your mouth is dry, or if your muscles are sore or cramping.

As a precautionary measure, it is a good idea to make sure your diet is rich in potassium while you are on a diuretic. High levels of potassium can be found in milk; in vegetables, such as raw carrots, lentils, lima beans, navy beans, and tomatoes; and in fruits—peaches, bananas, citrus fruits, and dried fruits such as apricots, figs, prunes, and raisins. Potassium is in good supply in beef, chicken, fish, liver, pork, almonds, peanut butter, all-bran cereals, breads, and crackers.

Remember: when you take drugs, you have to anticipate their effect on any product of the reproductive system, most particularly a fetus. Diuretics are meant to be taken right before the menstrual flow begins, something that will not happen if you are pregnant. So we must caution you once again. If you are trying to to get pregnant, these drugs can cause problems. Thiazides can damage an embryo in its earliest days. Furosemide has caused fetal abnormalities when fed to pregnant laboratory animals. And the manufacturer of the popular American brand, Lasix, states clearly that the drug should be given to women of childbearing age only when it is crucial to save their lives.

Vitamin B-6. One treatment for PMS that may work for you is pyridoxine, commonly known as vitamin B-6. This is actually not a drug but a water-soluble vitamin that can be excreted by your body if you take too much. Some women claim it provides relief from depression, aggression, and headaches.

This vitamin treatment may take a few months to take effect, and you may have to try gradually increasing the number of milligrams until you find the amount that's right for you. But don't take more that two hundred milligrams a day, or you may find yourself suffering from gastric acidity. If doses up to two hundred milligrams daily don't work, then vitamin B-6 probably is not a treatment that will help you.

Women who say B-6 works for them report they are free of monthly headaches and even depression. And some women who have taken vitamin B-6 for nine months and then stopped taking it say their symptoms did not return. Of course, it is important to check with your physician before you start any vitamin regimen.

Synthetic progesterone. One of the synthetic progesterones used for the treatment of PMS is dydrogesterone. It resembles natural progesterone and has been used successfully at St. Thomas' Hospital in London in treating both water retention and psychological symptoms. Three-quarters of the women treated were either completely relieved of symptoms or felt so much better they could cope with whatever discomfort that remained.

Dydrogesterone (Duphaston) can be administered orally in doses of ten milligrams twice a

When you take drugs you have to anticipate their effect on the reproductive system.

day to start. It is taken from Day 12 to Day 28 of the cycle. Sometimes forty milligrams a day is prescribed at first; the dosage is then reduced. The treatment time usually is six to nine months.

Among the side effects observed at St. Thomas' Hospital were mild nausea, breast tenderness in women who had no premenstrual tenderness before, and recurrence of breast tenderness in women who were all too familiar with it. There were also some changes in the menstrual cycle. Dydrogesterone is a hormone, so the cautions in taking any hormone medication should be observed. At the present time no tests link dydrogesterone to cancer.

Oral contraceptives. Just as the birth control pill has been prescribed as a treatment for painful periods, it has been used to treat PMS. The pill suppresses ovulation, and few if any women who do not ovulate suffer from premenstrual syndrome. However, the pill brings with its contraceptive bonus a number of side effects. Some women suffer from depression when on the pill and others get headaches—even when they have never previously suffered from those symptoms premenstrually. Anyone who gets migraine headaches on the pill should stop taking it. The headache-pill combination is associated with stroke in pill users, especially those who smoke.

Talk to your physician about your premenstrual symptoms. Together you can map out the strategy to bring you relief.

CHAPTER FIVE

RELIEF IS JUST A STRETCH AWAY

Ever since you donned your first pair of sneakers, you've probably been told that exercise is good for you. Your physical education teachers may well have announced that exercise was especially good for you at *that* time of the month. They may have urged you, or ordered you, to get into your shorts and out onto the gym floor. But a few laps around the track did not make you feel better. Instead, you probably moved like a teen-age Quasimodo.

Depending upon how bad your menstrual cramps are, or how uncomfortable premenstrual syndrome makes you, you might want to take it easy at this time of the month. While you are resting, however, there are a number of ways you can deal with the abdominal cramps or the lower back pain that may accompany your periods. Try applying heat. The use of a hot water bottle or heating pad may be a folk remedy, but it also makes medical sense. Heat can

help ease those painful uterine spasms. Sometimes massaging your stomach area and back with deep-heating creams or oils that are sold over the counter can bring relief, too.

If you can neither take to your bed nor apply heating creams or oils that may give off a pungent smell, try a light, fingertip massage alone. This won't make your stomach or your back much warmer, but it may be slightly numbing.

Another warm approach to menstrual pain is total immersion: in other words, a hot bath. Aromatic bath oils and soothing herbs that fill the air with fragrance are refreshing and relaxing for some women, nauseating for others. If smells make your stomach flip, keep them out of your bath water. You can stay in a hot tub for as long as you find it comfortable and helpful; just make sure the water is not too hot. Excessive heat can cause nausea and fainting spells. Later in this chapter, we will describe several exercises you can do while you are lying in the tub.

In addition to applying heat externally, you may get some relief from internal heat. Hot liquids—clear soups, broths, and herbal teas—can have a calming effect. If you find a little alcohol helps you relax, try hot tea with some whiskey or rum. But be cautious: just like too much heat, too much liquor can make some women nauseous and dizzy.

These ways of dealing with the discomforts of premenstrual syndrome and menstrual pain, however, are really stopgap measures to get you through a few painful hours or days. For a more permanent solution, condition your body while you are feeling good.

Exercise can help you cope with menstrual discomfort in a number of ways. One of the things we have learned from the school of prepared childbirth sometimes known as the La-Maze method (after a French pioneer of the technique) is that a muscle—in this case, the uterus—that is relaxed will cause less discomfort than a muscle that's clenched. Many women who suffer every month become apprehensive as their period approaches and involuntarily tense up, gritting their psychological teeth to deal with the upcoming pain. This tenses muscles, too, which only makes things worse. Relief may be a stretch away.

Shallow, panicked breathing deprives the body of oxygen, which causes numbness, tingling in the extremeties, and dizziness. The exercises that follow are aimed at encouraging slow, deep breathing, so that you can get much-needed oxygen to your uterus and other muscles, helping you feel relaxed, indulged, calm, and fit.

These exercises may also help banish those aches in the back, legs, thighs, and ankles that are often caused by fluid retention. And they can help get rid of extra fluid by stimulating your circulation.

For best results, exercise every day. Be careful not to overexert yourself, especially at the beginning. Pay attention to special physical conditions that may rule out some of the exercises—back problems, for example.

Once you've done the exercises, try lightly massaging the different sections of your body: face, head, neck and shoulders, back, legs, and ankles. You should feel as if you've been worked over by a skilled masseuse. Actually, if you have the time and the money, a professional massage can ease premenstrual tension.

The following chart can be used as a quick reference to help you determine which exercises will work best to ease your particular menstrual problems.

For Premenstrual Syndrome Sufferers

If You Have Menstrual Cramps

General Relaxation and Strengthening Exercises

1 Relaxation Breathing

Let us start with a simple exercise that will help you relax all the parts of your body.

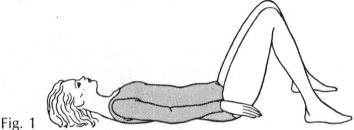

Fig. 1

Lie on your back on the floor or a bed. Bend your knees, placing your feet flat on the floor about a foot apart. Your arms should be at your sides and your shoulders flat. Relax your hands, Fig. 1.

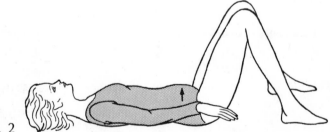

Fig. 2

Now, as you count to five, breathe in deeply through your nose. Let your abdomen and chest expand as they fill slowly with air. Imagine the air filling your head, neck, arms, and legs as well, replacing any tension that might be there, Fig. 2.

Relax all parts of your body as you breathe in a steady rhythm.

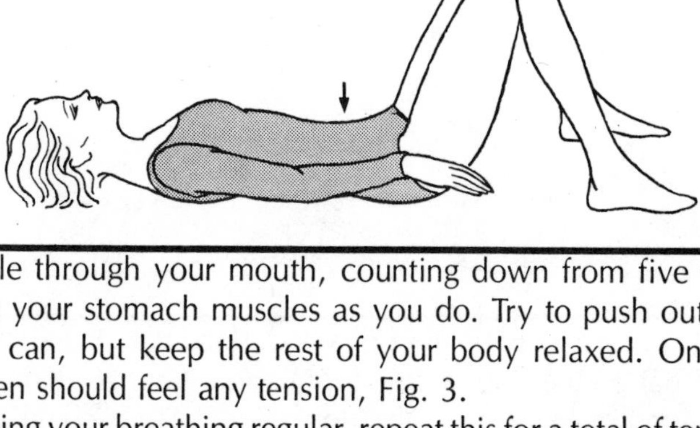

Fig. 3

Exhale through your mouth, counting down from five to one. Tighten your stomach muscles as you do. Try to push out all the air you can, but keep the rest of your body relaxed. Only your abdomen should feel any tension, Fig. 3.

Keeping your breathing regular, repeat this for a total of ten times. On days when you feel strong, you may want to count higher than five. Remember, this exercise is not an endurance test; it is designed to relax you and get you to breathe in a deep and regular manner.

Once you feel relaxed, you can move on to the next exercises.

2 Heads Up

This exercise will help strengthen your abdominal muscles and simultaneously begin to take some of the pressure off your back. Sagging stomach muscles put extra strain on your back, which causes pain. When your stomach muscles are strong, they help your back hold your body upright. They also keep your stomach flatter on the days just before your period.

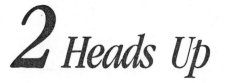

Fig. 1

Lie on your back on the floor or a bed. Bend your knees, placing your feet flat on the floor about a foot apart. Your arms should be at your sides, palms flat on the floor, Fig. 1. To a count of five, breathe in slowly through your nose, filling your abdomen and chest with air. Then open your mouth and exhale, counting down from five, contracting your abdomen and lifting your head as far off the pillow as you can. Keep your shoulders, arms, and hands relaxed

Always lower your head back down slowly and gently.

and uninvolved. They should not be used to push your head up. Only your head, neck, and stomach muscles should be working, Fig. 2.

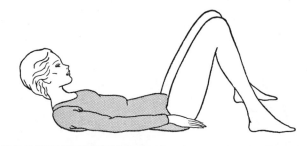

Fig. 2

At the highest point your head can reach, hold and count to five as you continue to breathe in and out.

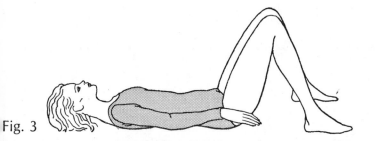

Fig. 3

At a point when you've exhaled, start to breathe in and slowly lower your head to the pillow or floor, Fig. 3.

If you suffer from a stiff neck or headaches around the time of your period, do not do this exercise if it makes the head pain worse.

3 Belly Book Bump

You'll need one prop for this stomach strengthener: a big, heavy, soft-covered book. If you live in a large metropolitan area, a telephone book should be perfect. If your information directory is skimpy, you can use a mail-order catalog. The big Sears book is fine.

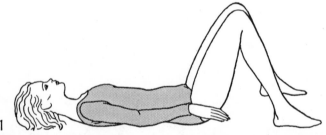

Fig. 1

Lie on your back on the floor or a bed. Bend your knees, placing your feet flat on the floor about shoulder width apart. Your arms should be at your sides, palms down, Fig. 1. Close your eyes if you like.

Keeping your stomach muscles loose, lightly bounce your belly up and in. While you are bouncing, take short, quick, panting breaths. Bounce and breathe for ten breaths. Do this series five times. You may want to rest between series; quick, shallow breathing can make you dizzy.

Now, put your heavy, soft-covered book across your abdomen.

Slight pressure may relieve uncomfortable spasms.

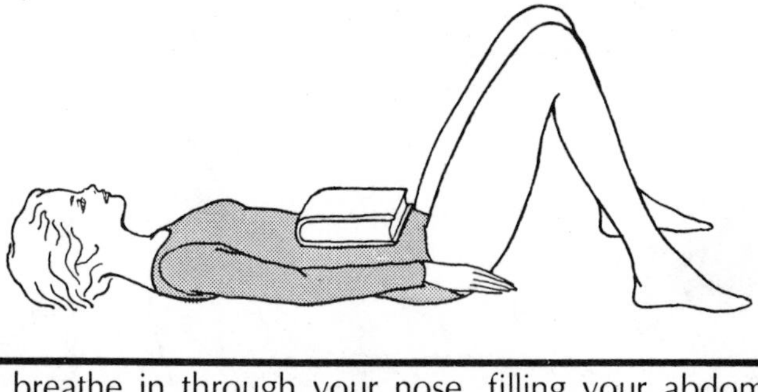

Fig. 2

Slowly breathe in through your nose, filling your abdomen and chest with air and pushing the book up. Hold for a count of five, Fig. 2.

On the count of six, begin to exhale slowly through your mouth, and let the book drop along with your stomach and chest. Contract your stomach muscles as much as you can. Hold for a count of five.

If you have bad cramps, you can substitute a heavy pillow for the book. But the book may be more effective, creating pressure that can relieve abdominal spasms.

4 Sitting Pull-Up

This exercise is a preliminary sit-up that offers some of the stomach strengthening benefits of the conventional sit-up without the strain. Like the previous exercises, it can be done in bed or on the floor. I prefer the floor: you have to work harder, and you'll get more out of it.

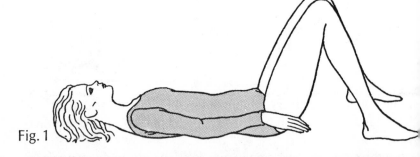

Fig. 1

Lie on your back with your knees bent and feet flat on the floor about a foot apart. Your arms should be at your sides with palms down, hands relaxed, Fig. 1.

Breathe in slowly through your nose, letting your torso fill with air. As you start to exhale through your mouth, grasp your right knee with both hands. Pull your knee toward your torso as you

You'll find this easier to do than a full sit-up, yet effective.

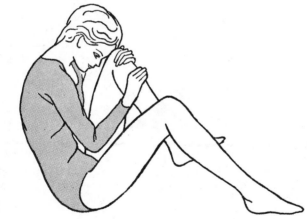

Fig. 2

rise to a sitting position. Hold for a count of five, Fig. 2.

Start to inhale slowly through your nose and release your knee. Let your leg and body drop slowly down to the floor.

Relax for a count of five.

Repeat the exercise, bringing your left knee to meet your chest as you exhale. Alternate legs, pulling each side up five times.

5 *Bridge to Relief*

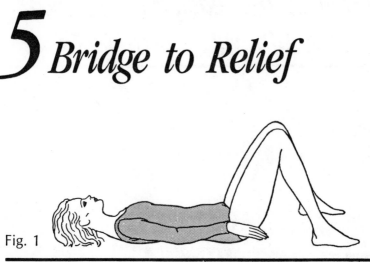

Fig. 1

Lie on your back on the floor or on a bed, keeping your knees bent, and place your feet flat on the floor about a foot in front of your buttocks. Your arms should be at your sides, palms down, Fig. 1.

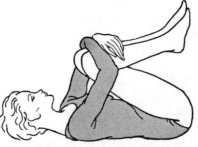

Fig. 2

    Raise your knees to your chest, grasping them with your arms. Pull them in toward your chest, Fig. 2. Now, release your legs and place your feet on the floor in their original position, Fig. 3.

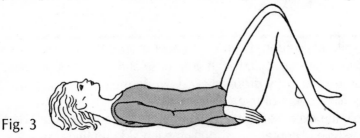

Fig. 3

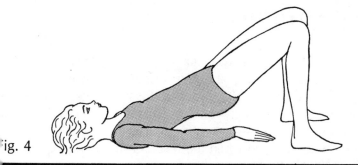

Fig. 4

Inhale through your nose. As you exhale slowly through your mouth, contract your abdominal muscles and lift your hips up off the floor, Fig. 4. This is your bridge to relief. Your body should be in a straight line from your knees to your neck, and you should feel a good stretch through your upper thighs and abdomen. Hold this position for a count of five to ten, depending upon how strong you are and how uncomfortable your midsection is.

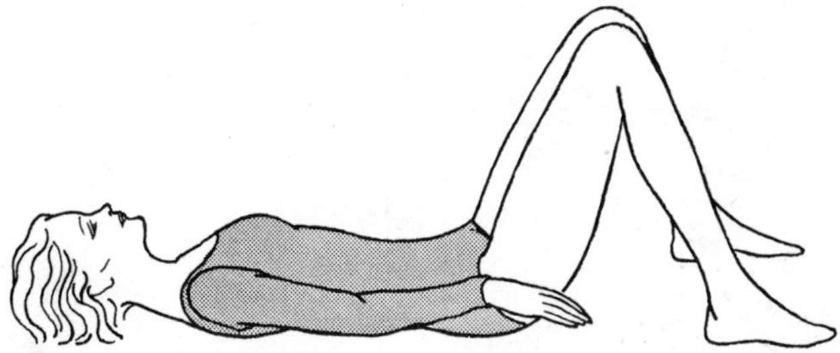

Fig. 5

Then slowly lower your torso to the floor, Fig. 5. Don't plop down. Instead, using the muscles of your thighs and stomach, lower yourself to the floor. Line your back up with the floor, making sure it's flat. Check by trying to slip one of your hands under the arch of your back. You want to eliminate any space there is.

Finally, raise your knees to your chest once again. Hug them with your arms. Let your legs go and return to starting position. Rest and breathe deeply. You may want to repeat this sequence several times. You'll find it very comforting.

6 Waterless Swim

This exercise will build up your stamina, firm the muscles in your abdomen and lower back, and help dispel the tension that can accompany your period. The Waterless Swim can get your entire body moving on a day when your menstrual flow is heavy but you have to get up and go.

Women who grew up when the first menstrual commandment was "Thou shalt not swim" may be surprised to learn that swimming is one of the best things you can do to relieve menstrual discomfort.

If you don't have year-round pool privileges or don't feel like getting wet, this dry swim comes close enough to swimming to tone the same muscles.

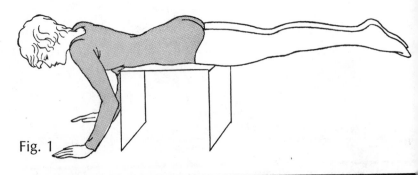

Fig. 1

You'll have to find a low, long stool or table. A sturdy coffee table will do, or a piano bench. It has to be strong enough to support the full weight of your body. A cushion across the top will make you and your hipbones more comfortable.

Lie on your stomach on the stool or table, with as much of your torso on the support as you can. Make sure your legs are free. Ideally, the support should stretch from just below your armpits to the top of your thighs, Fig. 1.

This exercise may prove difficult at first but it is worth the effort.

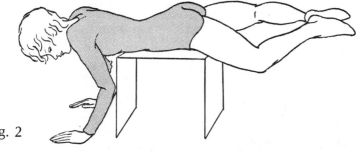

Fig. 2

For balance, put your hands down on the floor in front of you. Start with your legs together, stretched straight out behind you. In one continuous, fluid motion, bend your knees, pulling both feet in as close to your buttocks as you can, soles together, and kick your legs out straight again, Fig. 2. Do a kind of frog kick.

Continue this swimming kick for two minutes, keeping a smooth, easy rhythm. Music may help. As your muscle tone and stamina improve, increase your continuous swimming time to five minutes.

7 Dromedary Droop

Some women find that when they have menstrual cramps, they feel most comfortable on their hands and knees. During labor, when the uterus enlarges and contracts, throwing the uterus forward and off the backbone can ease discomfort. Most women in labor don't get down on their hands and knees; instead, they bend over, getting their heads lower than their bellies. This position makes them less uncomfortable. The same principle can work for a menstruating uterus.

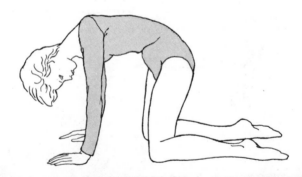

Fig. 1

Get down on all fours, either on the floor or on a bed. Place your palms flat on the floor, keeping your shoulders down and making your back straight, like a table.

Inhale slowly through your nose. Then, exhale through your mouth, forcing out all the air you can. Contract your abdominal muscles and hump your back like a camel. Tuck your head down so you are looking at your navel. Hold for a count of five, Fig.1.

Release and breathe in slowly through your nose. Flatten your

Try this if you are feeling pressure on your back coupled with menstrual cramps.

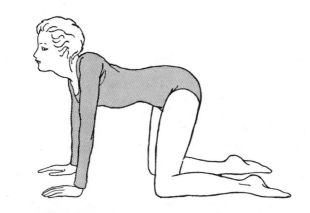

Fig. 2

back once again and lift your head until you are looking straight ahead. Hold this position for a count of five, Fig. 2.

Repeat this exercise six times.

If you are feeling really terrible and it is too difficult for you, try this. Get on your knees and place your forearms on the floor, each hand grasping the opposite forearm. Let your head drop all the way down to rest on your folded arms. You may want to put a pillow under your arms. Rest in this position.

8 Bow and Stretch

When you are up to a little motion, try this stretch. A curled-up position can help diminish the pain, and stretching can bring you more relief than just lying still.

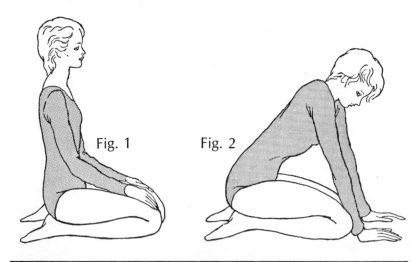

Fig. 1   Fig. 2

Kneel on a carpeted floor, knees together. Sit back on your heels. The tops of your feet should be against the floor, Fig. 1.

Bend forward with your arms straight and palms out. Place your palms on the floor, Fig. 2. Slide your hands along the floor until

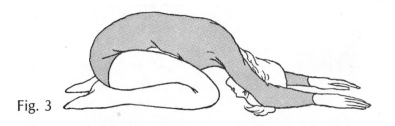

Fig. 3

your forehead touches the floor, Fig. 3. Your rib cage should be lifted and free. Gently breathe in and out, relax, close your eyes, and stay in this position for as long as you like.

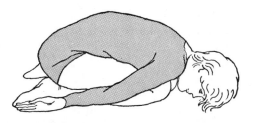

Fig. 4

When you are rested and relaxed, slide your arms back until your hands rest alongside your feet, palms up. Keep your chest on your knees, Fig. 4.

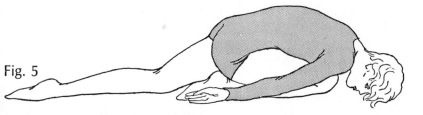

Fig. 5

Now, move the weight of your body so it rests on your right leg and move your left leg straight out back, Fig. 5. You may waver a little as you readjust your balance. Hold this stretched-back position for a few minutes. Then pull your left leg in under your chest once again.

Repeat this stretch with the right leg, your torso weight shifted to your left foot. Hold this position. Tuck this leg back under you again.

With pauses and rests in between, repeat this part of the exercise five times, alternating the stretched positions with the tucked.

9 Chair Relief

If you get dizzy at any time during this exercise, stop. Women with high blood pressure should check with their doctors before they proceed. If your blood pressure is normal, you should realize that as you get stronger, the dizziness will decrease.

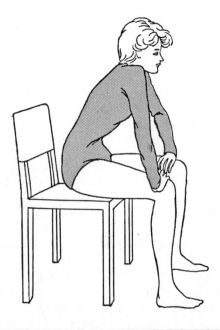

Fig. 1

Sit about halfway back on a low-back chair. Put your feet flat on the floor, about a chair width apart. Place your hands on your thighs slightly above your knees and spread your fingers out comfortably. Lean your body forward just a bit, raising your shoulders toward your ears, Fig. 1. Keep your torso in a line from the tip of

For relieving menstrual discomfort when you are at the office...

your head to your tailbone. Don't slouch or fall forward too far.

Inhale as much as you can through your nose. Now, exhale through your open mouth, emptying your chest and abdomen of all the air you can. Contract your stomach muscles and pull them in and under your rib cage as much as possible. Your goal is a concave stomach, Fig. 2. Hold this position for a few seconds; then release.

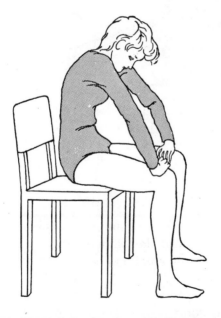

Fig. 2

Even after you pull in as far as you can, some belly may be left behind. Put one hand on the flesh and gently move it in the direction of the muscles. With time and work, your belly may follow by itself, or you may have to lose some weight.

This is a fine conditioning exercise and can relieve discomfort.

10 Rocking Dive

Rocking is an instinctive human motion when we are hurting. Parents rock their babies and we rock ourselves. Rocking can bring temporary relief from menstrual cramps, soothing abdominal spasms.

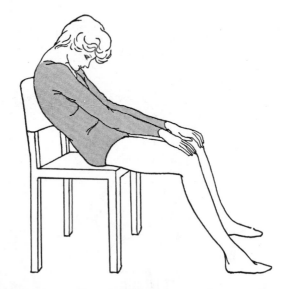

Fig. 1

Sit about halfway back in a comfortable low-back chair. You can use a rocking chair if you like. Stretch your legs out in front of you with your knees slightly apart and bent. Keep your feet flat on the floor.

Lean backward so your back touches the chair. Drop your arms down comfortably onto your legs or onto the chair arms. Your body should be concave, and you should feel like you are slouching in the chair, Fig. 1.

Slowly breathe in through your nose and fill your abdomen and chest with air. Draw your hands together into a diver's position and raise your arms to shoulder level. Exhale slowly through your

Another easy office exercise to help relieve menstrual discomfort.

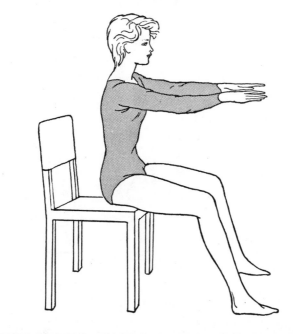

Fig. 2

mouth, contract your abdominal muscles, and pull yourself to an erect sitting position, back straight, Fig. 2. Hold this position for a slow count of three. Inhale and slowly drop back to your original, curved position. Your buttocks should remain still throughout the exercise.

Rock forward and back smoothly. Don't jerk yourself forward and then fall back. Your abdominal muscles should control each motion. At the end of one set, relax. Stretch your fingers. Rotate your shoulders.

Gradually work up to ten sets. Take it easy at first, especially if your stomach is soft and weak.

11 *Chair Cheer*

If you are doing this exercise in your office remember, it is fairly dramatic and will attract more attention than the previous ones. Close your door if you are at work, or prepare for an audience.

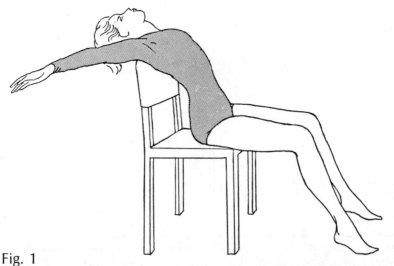

Fig. 1

Once again, sit about halfway back in a low-back chair. Bend your knees, keeping them far apart, and put your feet flat on the floor. Raise your arms above your head in a Y-position, and stretch your arms, upper torso, and head as far back as you can, Fig. 1. You should be staring at the ceiling. Breathe in slowly through your mouth. Fill up with air.

Now, begin to exhale through your mouth and swing your arms down and together, contract your abdominal muscles, and let your head drop down through your legs. With your arms, stretch and

If this exercise makes you feel dizzy, don't do it.

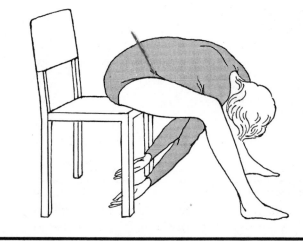

Fig. 2

reach along the floor toward the back of the chair, Fig. 2. Hold this position for a slow count of five.

On six, begin to unfold. Inhale through your nose and pull up with your head. Let your arms follow as you return to your original position. Keep your buttocks on the chair and your feet flat on the floor.

Your goal is to swing your body smoothly. Stretch only as far as you comfortably can. With practice, you will get more limber.

Repeat this exercise five to ten times.

12 Ankle Roll

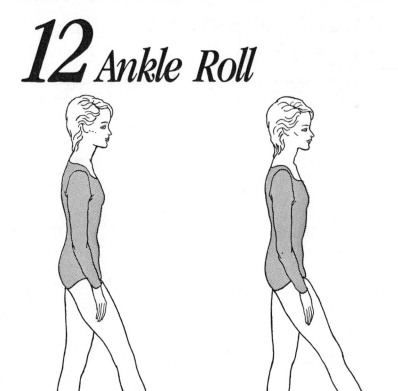

Fig. 1   Fig. 2

Stand up straight with your feet slightly apart, arms at your sides, resting on your hip bones. Keeping the leg straight and the foot relaxed, lift your right leg approximately six inches off the floor, Fig. 1. Flex your right foot as much as you can, toes pointing toward the ceiling, Fig. 2. Hold that flexed, extended position for a slow count of five. Keeping your leg off the floor, let your foot and ankle relax. Hold your foot in this relaxed position for a count of five. Return it to the standing position.

Repeat with left foot and leg.

After doing the exercise with each foot, bend your knees and shake out your legs and feet.

Return to the standing position and repeat the set.

13 Arm Swings

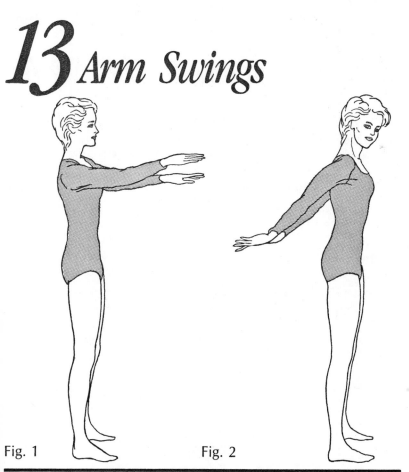

Fig. 1   Fig. 2

Stand up with your feet slightly apart and knees and back straight. Let your arms hang loosely at your sides, keeping your shoulders down and relaxed. Breathe in slowly through your nose and slowly raise your arms out to your sides until they are shoulder height, palms down. Make sure your shoulders are still down and relaxed. They should not creep up toward your ears. Hold this position for a slow count of five. Exhale through your mouth and swing your arms in front of you, scissoring your right arm over your left, Fig. 1, then swing them back behind you as far as they can go, Fig. 2. Breathing through your mouth, repeat these swings ten times. Alternate left over right arm, then right over left. Keep your elbows straight. Your middle back tension will be gone.

14 Up Against the Wall

Right before your period, or during it, you may feel as if you are dragging your midsection along behind you. This exercise will help make the lower back more flexible and strengthen a weak stomach. An exaggerated swayback not only makes your bottom appear bigger than it is, but can also lead to difficulty in moving and painful bowel problems. Those conditions will be with you all month long; menstrual complications will only make them worse. Investing just fifteen minutes a day in exercises that strengthen your abdomen and improve your posture can pay off in a pain-free, flexible existence.

Do not do either version of the following exercise if it causes pain in your back.

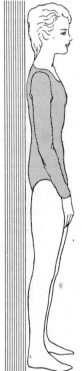

Fig. 1

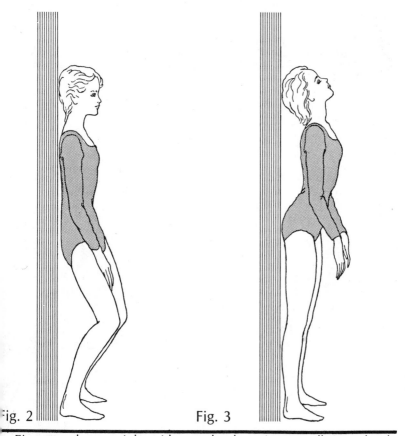

Fig. 2   Fig. 3

First, stand up straight with your back against a wall. Your heels should touch the wall, too, Fig, 1.

Contract the muscles in your buttocks and bend your knees until your back and waist are flat against the wall.

Now, get your abdomen involved. Pull your bottom in hard, and roll your pelvis and hips forward, Fig. 2. To do this correctly, you have to contract both the buttocks and the abdominal muscles. Exhale to the count of five as you contract. Then hold for a few more counts. As you get stronger, increase the holding time.

Next, start to inhale, straightening your legs and arching your back so much that it feels like you are almost sitting on the wall, Fig. 3. Flex yourself from the flat to arched positions as quickly and as smoothly as you can. Begin with five repetitions and build up to ten.

15 Pelvic Tilt

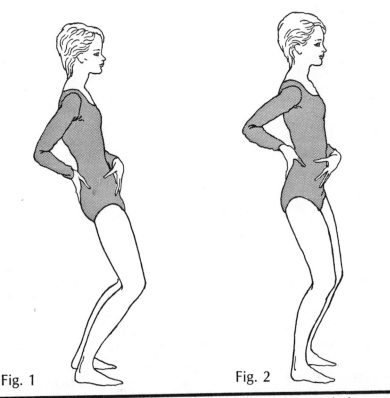

Fig. 1   Fig. 2

Once you get the feeling of Exercise, 14 you can work the same muscles standing away from a wall or even sitting down. Place one hand on your back and the other on your lower abdomen to help push you back and forth. Or, hold onto your waist and feel your hips and pelvis shift back and forth, Figs. 1 and 2.

Your back will be more flexible, your abdomen stronger, and your cramps less severe.

16 *The Prayer*

Stand comfortably erect with your feet slightly apart. Inhale slowly through your nose and bring your arms up until they are parallel to the floor.

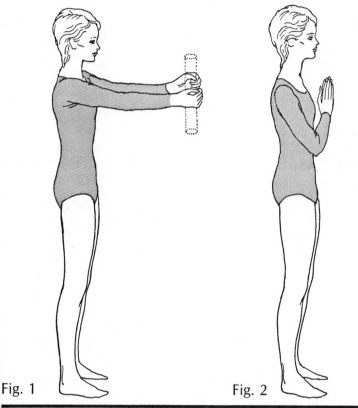

Fig. 1   Fig. 2

grasping an imaginary vertical pole in front of you, Fig. 1.

Begin to exhale through your mouth and gradually loosen your hands from the "pole," leaving them gently together. Draw your elbows in to your sides so that you are in a "praying" position, Fig. 2.

Repeat this three times.

The Prayer will get oxygen into your system, relieving tension.

17 *Tiptoe and Drop*

Don't go so high on your toes that you lose your balance.

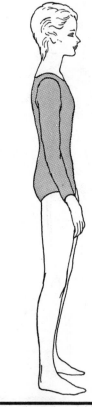

Fig. 1

Assume a comfortable standing position. Your feet should be about fifteen inches apart, your arms hanging loosely at your sides, Fig.1.

Breathe in slowly through your nose and simultaneously raise your arms as you lift yourself up onto your toes, Fig. 2.

Hold yourself in this position for a count of five. You may have to adjust your position to balance yourself.

Next, exhale through your mouth, contract your abdominal mus-

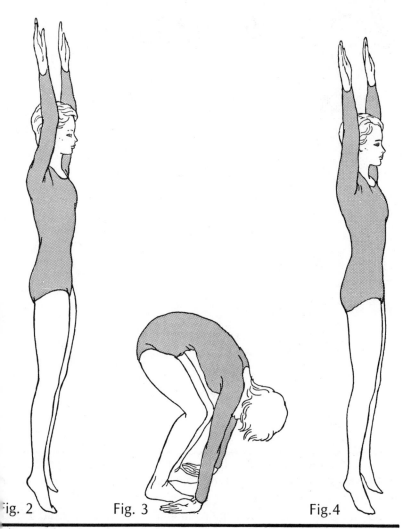

Fig. 2   Fig. 3   Fig.4

cles, and swing down into a semi-crouch position. Let your feet drop down flat onto the floor, bend your knees, and swing your arms down so that the backs of your hands rest against the floor, Fig. 3. Hold this position for a count of five.

Inhale slowly through your mouth and gradually return yourself to the tiptoe, arms-up position, Fig. 4.

Repeat this exercise six times.

18 *Back Stretch*

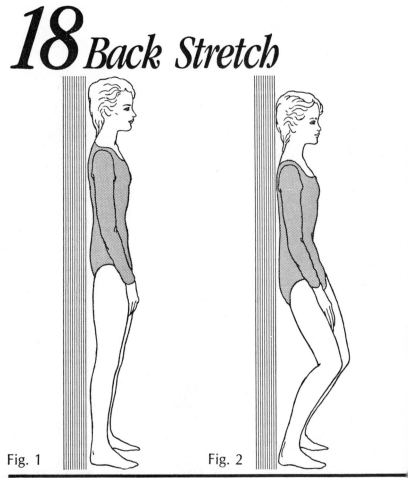

Fig. 1   Fig. 2

The Back Stretch can be helpful for a number of back problems. But if you already have back trouble, ask your physician whether this exercise is good for you.

Stand up with your back against a wall. Your heels should touch the wall, too, Fig. 1. Bend your knees as far as you must to eliminate the empty space between your lower back and the wall. Let your arms and hands hang loosely at your sides, Fig. 2.

Pull your abdominal muscles in, keeping your pelvis tucked under. Slowly inch your body up the wall, keeping your back flat the entire time. Your goal is to keep your back flat and completely against the wall while you move your calves in closer and closer

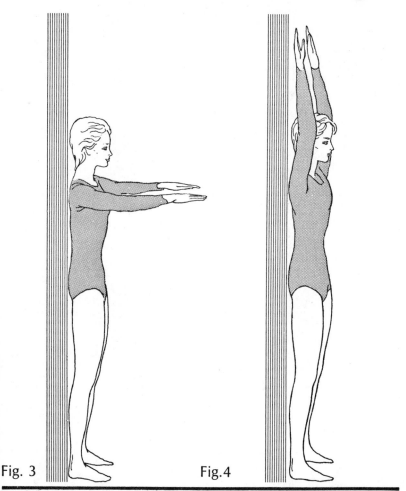

Fig. 3   Fig.4

until they touch the wall. Don't be discouraged; it may be months until you are stretched out enough to do it. Keep your breathing deep and regular during this exercise.

Hold your final position and stretch your arms out together in front of you, Fig. 3. Slowly raise them until they are overhead, Fig. 4. Aim at bringing them back, still straight, to touch the wall while you keep your head, back, calves, and heels against the wall.

Work every day to move your arms higher and higher. This lifts your entire rib cage, letting your chest cavity fill with air and toning your pelvic girdle.

19 *Say Ha*

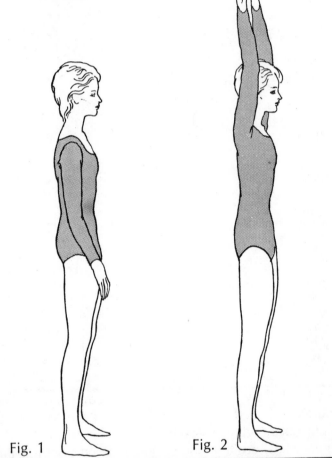

Fig. 1   Fig. 2

Assume a comfortable standing position with feet slightly apart, Fig. 1. As you breathe in slowly through your nose, raise your arms straight up over your head. Stretch up and reach for the ceiling with your fingertips, Fig. 2. Hold for a count of five. Then, on the count of six, swing your arms and your upper torso forward in one fluid motion. Let your body bend comfortably at the waist, Fig. 3. As you swing and bend, force your breath out of your mouth in

Bend your knees if your hands don't touch the floor.

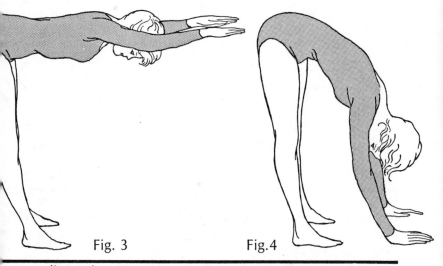

Fig. 3   Fig.4

one explosive *ha*. Continue expelling all the air from your lungs, panting *ha* again and again, until your lungs are empty.

When the air is all expelled, let yourself hang down limply like a rag doll, and swing gently back and forth from the waist, if you choose, Fig. 4. Finally, inhale slowly, lift your torso up until it is straight, and stretch your arms up overhead. Repeat this exercise two times.

20 Relaxtic Band

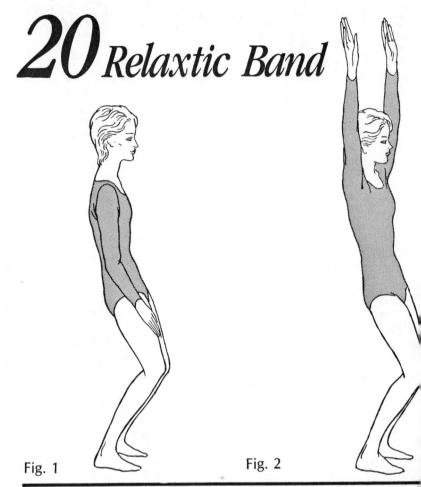

Fig. 1

Fig. 2

Stand up straight with your feet about shoulder width apart. Bend your knees slightly and tuck your buttocks and hips under you. Contract your abdominal muscles. Let your arms hang loosely at your sides, Fig. 1.

Slowly raise your arms out, palms down, then bring them up until your fingertips are pointing toward the ceiling, Fig. 2. Now, stretch your right arm up as far as you can, without lifting your right foot off the floor, Fig. 3. Relax. Stretch your right arm up four times. Then repeat with your left arm.

Try pretending you are grabbing for a gymnastic ring suspended on a strong elastic strap. You want to reach up and pull it down.

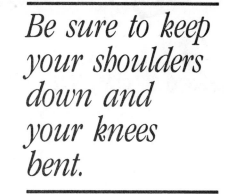

Be sure to keep your shoulders down and your knees bent.

Fig. 3

Fig. 4

Pretend that the strong elastic is giving you a lot of resistance. Reach and pull firmly.

After you have stretched both arms, let them drop down and at the same time allow your upper body to fall forward. Bend your knees. Relax your arms, hands, shoulders, neck, and head, Fig. 4. Let gravity help pull you down. Pretend you are a puppet hung by a string attached just below your belt. Your hands should touch your toes, or be close to them. Swing back and forth on your ''string.'' Gently move all your joints until you feel loose.

Slowly curl up to a standing position.

Repeat this exercise five times.

21 Shoulder Lifts

You can do this exercise either standing up or sitting in a straight-back chair.

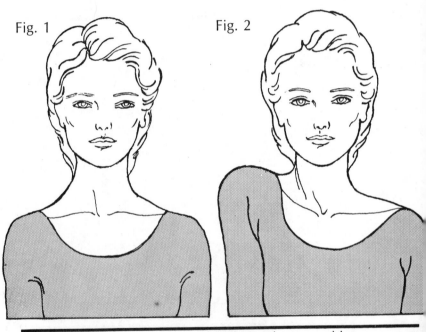

Fig. 1   Fig. 2

Hold your torso erect, your head straight up, and let your arms hang loosely at your sides, Fig. 1.

Without moving your head, slowly increase the muscle tension in right arm and lift your shoulder as close to your ear as you can, Fig. 2. Hold it there for a count of five. On six, drop your shoulder, quickly releasing the tension. Let it go with a downward thrust.

Relax for a count of five, then repeat this exercise on the left side. Alternate the tension-release from right to left.

Finally, tense and lift both shoulders simultaneously. Hold for a count of five and drop them quickly.

22 *Shoulder Circles*

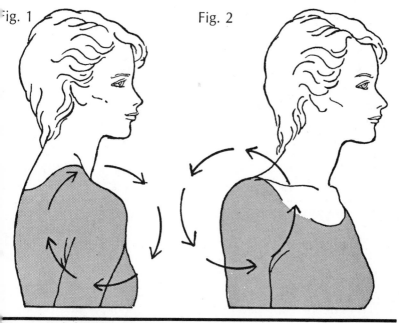

Fig. 1   Fig. 2

Sit or stand, letting your arms hang loosely at your sides. Begin to move your right shoulder in a full forward circle, Fig. 1. Start by moving it forward and toward the center of your chest. From this forward-center position, move your shoulder up to your ear and then back and in, pushing toward your spine. Now, return your shoulder to its starting position. Repeat this forward circle three times, then reverse direction, Fig. 2. Make three backward circles before you switch to your left side.

After you've loosened each side individually, circle both shoulders forward together, then back. Your shoulder sockets should feel wobbly and loose. Your head may feel that way, too.

23 Head Drop

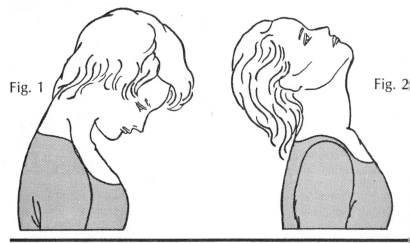

Fig. 1   Fig. 2

Do this exercise to reduce tension in the neck area.

Either sit up straight in a chair or sit on the floor in a cross-legged position. Let your arms and hands rest loosely on the chair arms or on your knees.

Let your head fall forward, Fig. 1. Do not jerk it, but let it loll. Instead of bending forward from your midsection, bend from your neck so you feel a pull along your spinal cord. Let gravity help you. Your head is heavy. Feel it pull you down. Hold this stretched position for a count of five.

Now, as if you were a puppet with a guide string attached to the front of your chin, pull your head up slowly until your face and chin are facing the ceiling, Fig. 2. Don't strain yourself, but feel the long pull along the front of your neck. Hold that position for a count of five.

Gradually return your head to an erect position. Relax. Repeat this exercise three times. Each time you do it, you may feel your head and neck stretching farther forward and back.

24 Head Roll

Head rolls will not only help work out monthly tensions, but can help you gain full flexibility in the neck area.

The best place to do this exercise is on the floor in a cross-legged position, but if you'd rather not, sit in an armchair and tuck your legs into a cross-legged position.

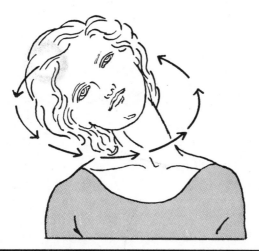

Hold onto your ankles with both hands and sit tall. Lean back ever so slightly and let your head flop back a bit. Relax your head and neck.

Keep your shoulders down during this exercise. Now, roll your head slowly and gently from the back to the left and all around the front in a clockwise position. Then reverse, and circle your head counterclockwise.

Stop if you become dizzy. Try to do a little more tomorrow. You may find you can't make a full circle, or that your neck cracks as you turn. Move through those spots slowly and carefully. With consistent exercise, you will come full circle.

25 *Facial Massage*

Women who suffer from premenstrual syndrome feel like they are getting a cold when they are actually getting their periods. Fluids and pressure can build up, causing sinuslike pain and headaches.

When you are feeling all filled up with fluid, turning on a humidifier may bring some relief. Or, try taking a hot, steamy bath.

The following facial exercises can be done almost anywhere, but they are especially nice to do in the tub. If you don't feel like taking a bath, sit on the floor in a straight-back cross-legged position for this massage, or sit relaxed in a chair.

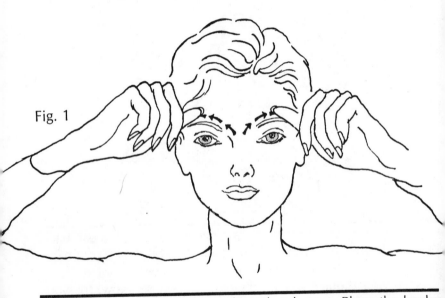

Fig. 1

Form your hands into loose fists, thumbs out. Place the backs of your thumbs over your eyebrows so that the tips are almost touching and they point toward the center of your forehead, nails against your face. Using long, smooth strokes, move your thumbs out toward your hairline and down along your temples, Fig. 1. Return your thumbs to your eyebrows and repeat this motion six times.

This provides soothing relief for facial tension anytime.

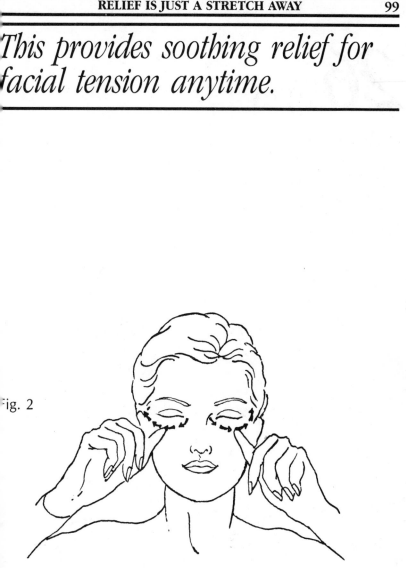

Fig. 2

On the sixth arc, continue the circle until your thumbs rest below your eyes, on either side of your nose. Gently massage the area under your eyes, moving out toward the temples again, Fig. 2. Repeat six times.

Remember: the skin under your eyes is especially delicate. Be gentle. To make the massage smoother, apply a light cream. Keep away from anything highly aromatic, if you are sensitive to smells.

26 *Eyes Up*

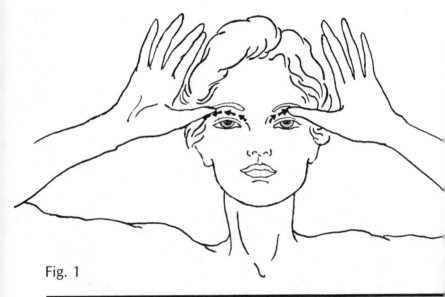

Fig. 1

Remain seated, either in a straight-back cross-legged position or in a chair. Open your hands and place the backs of your thumbs gently on the top of your eyelids, pinkies pointing out and up. Slowly and lightly slide your thumbs across the top of your eyelids out toward your temples, Fig. 1. Return your thumbs to their original position near your nose and repeat the outward stroke six times.

Now place the pads of your index fingers under your eyes, on

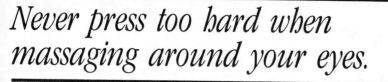

Never press too hard when massaging around your eyes.

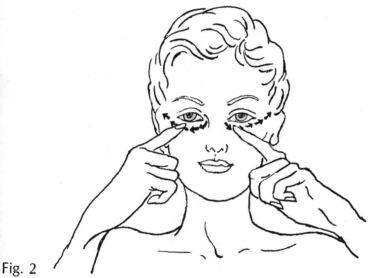

Fig. 2

the lower rim of the eye sockets. Gently slide your fingers out to the corners of your eyes and up toward the temples, Fig. 2. Keep your hands loose and relaxed. You may want to shake them between strokes to get rid of any tension. Repeat the motion six times.

Be very careful not to exert too much pressure around your eyes. If the skin feels dry or if you are tugging it as you massage, apply a light cream or lotion.

27 Look Around

You can look around during this eye exercise, or you can keep your eyes closed.

Hold your head up and still. Let your face muscles relax. If you are doing this exercise with your eyes open, close them after each step. Do each step three times, or any number you are comfortable with.

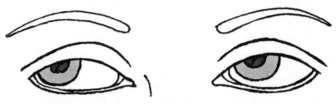

1. Look straight ahead. Slowly move your eyes as far to the right as you can, Fig. 1. Feel your eye muscles stretch. Return your eyes to the center. Repeat the same stretch on the left side. Hold each smooth stretch for a slow count of three. Close your eyes and relax.

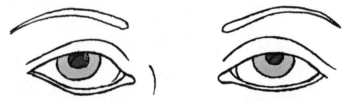

2. Look straight ahead. Slowly move your eyes up in your head until you are looking at the ceiling, Fig. 2. Return your eyes to the front.

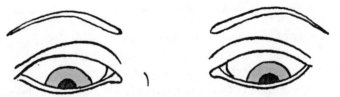

3. Now, look down, Fig. 3. Try to see your lips. Return your eyes to the front. Close your eyes and relax.

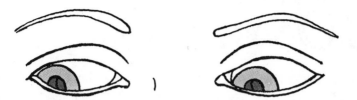

4. Look straight ahead. Move your eyes to the lower right, Fig. 4. Look straight once again. Now, look to the upper left. Return your eyes to the center. Close your eyes and rest.

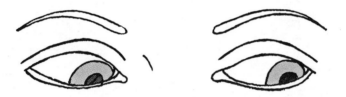

5. Look straight ahead. Move your eyes to the lower left, Fig. 5. Look straight once again. Now, look to the upper right. Return your eyes to the center. Close your eyes and rest.

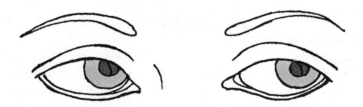

6. Look straight ahead. First, look down. Now, roll your eyes in a clockwise direction, continuing around the entire circle, Fig. 6. When your eyes come fully around, reverse the circle and move them counterclockwise. When they are centered again, close your eyes. Squeeze the lids together very tightly. Blink your eyelids as fast as you can. Finally, close your eyes gently and relax.

28 *Soak Down*

The following two exercises are designed as immersion therapy, using hot water, a relaxant that comes out of your tap. The first is really not an exercise at all, but a spine relaxer.

For the first water exercise, you will need two towels. Sink one onto the bottom of the tub. It will work as a skid mat and keep you from sliding. Fold the second towel to use as a head pillow.

Run the tub water as hot as you can enjoy.

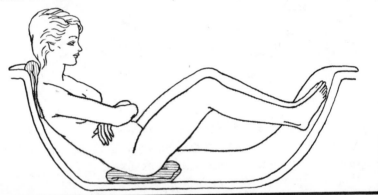

Slip down into the water and stretch your legs out. You want your back totally immersed in water, so you may have to prop your feet on the rim of the tub.

Now, slowly inhale through your nose to the count of five. Exhale through your mouth to another count of five. Fill up with air as completely as you can and then push out all that you've inhaled. While you breathe you should mentally check that you are completely relaxed. There should be no strain or discomfort in any part of your body.

After several minutes of concentrated deep breathing, relax. Let the water work on loosening your spine. When the water cools off, you may run more hot water into the tub. Soak as long as you like.

While you are in the water, salvage a bit of energy and try the next exercise, the Tub Tuck.

29 Tub Tuck

The Tub Tuck can help increase your blood circulation and strengthen your back.

Remove the towel from behind your head from the previous exercise, the Soak Down. Leave the towel you are using as a skid mat in place. You don't want to slip totally down into the water.

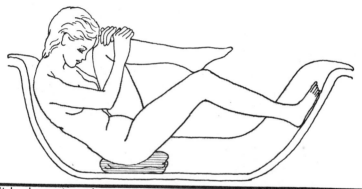

Slide down into the water so your back is completely immersed. Brace your left foot against the far edge of the tub above the water line, or against the wall.

Breathe in through your nose to the count of five. As you begin to exhale through your mouth, grasp your right knee with both hands and pull it in toward your chest and tucked-in head. Hold for a count of five. Then breathe in slowly once again, releasing your leg. Repeat this with your left leg, using your right as a brace. Do the exercise six times with each leg. At the end, bring both legs to your chest, and then stretch them straight out. Relax.

For the best results keep the water at a temperature right for you.

CHAPTER SIX

CAN I GO SWIMMING...AND ANSWERS TO OTHER MENSTRUAL QUESTIONS

Can I go swimming when I menstruate?

Yes. The old husbands' tale said that if you swam or took a bath when you menstruated, you risked catching cold. That's not so. In fact, swimming, an excellent all-round conditioner, is good for most women during their periods. Instead of confining yourself to the Waterless Swim exercise on page 68 to relieve discomfort, try the same motions in the water. Many women stop flowing when they take a bath or swim, so don't be surprised if the tampon you inserted right before diving in is hardly stained when you change after being in the water.

What happens if I have sexual intercourse during my period?

It is perfectly safe to have sex during your period, but don't make the mistake of thinking that you can't get pregnant at that time. You can. Pregnancy is more of a possibility in the first few days of your monthly cycle, just when you've started to bleed, than it is in the last few days of the cycle, just before you bleed. Sexual intercourse during menstruation is not painful for most women, but those who get cramps may have tenderness and find penetration uncomfortable.

Is exercise harmful during menstruation?

Exercise is good for you at all times, including during menstruation. It helps relax your muscles and can relieve your discomfort. But don't do exercises that make you feel worse and don't push yourself beyond your personal limits. If you can't manage any of the exercises suggested in this book, you may want to try sitting with your feet up when you are bleeding very heavily.

Does my period make me break out?

It certainly can. Women who are susceptible to acne often find the changes in the body's hormonal levels a week to ten days before menstruation causes their skin to erupt. Some women take the birth control pill to suppress their natural hormonal changes. Others follow their dermatologist's advice and apply topical medications or take a low dosage of tetracycline—an antibiotic that sometimes helps keep acne under control.

Do irregular periods mean something is wrong with my body?

No. The cycle-controlling center in the hypothalmus at the base of the brain is extraordinarily sensitive and easily affected by any number of factors, from a change in diet to a change in the weather to going up in an airplane to major emotional upsets. In fact, irregularity may be perfectly normal for you. The menstrual cycle is regulated by very delicate and intricate machinery, yet people expect it to be the same month after month. What is amazing is not that women are irregular, but that they are ever regular.

By what age should a young woman get her first period?

Girls start to menstruate anywhere from age nine to age fifteen, with the average age now being 12.3 years old.

One signal that a girl may soon start to menstruate is a growth spurt. This can be caused by the estrogen that her body begins to produce before she starts to menstruate. When the spurt slows down, menstruation begins.

If the first period doesn't show up by age sixteen, a complete endocrinological work-up may be in order.

What does it mean if I don't menstruate?

If you have never menstruated, you have what is called primary amenorrhea. The most common cause of delayed menstruation is constitutionally delayed puberty. Somewhere in your family background, you may find a mother, father, or more distant relative who had a very late physical development. Remember that girls undergoing strenuous physical training often start menstruating much later than the average age. But do take the time to consult a doctor.

What does it mean if I used to menstruate and don't anymore?

If you have menstruated and then stop, you have what is called secondary amenorrhea. The most frequent cause of this is pregnancy. The second is stress, often brought on by extreme swings in weight. A dramatic gain or loss of pounds can have an immediate effect on the cycling center in the brain. When a young woman comes to see me and complains that her periods have stopped, I generally ask her if she started a diet around the time of her last period. If the answer is yes, I try to establish how strict her diet still is. For example, is she still weighing her food? In cases of the starvation disease anorexia nervosa, stringent dieting may upset the delicate cycling center and stop the period even before weight loss is extreme. A third reason some periods stop is drugs. About twenty years ago the phenothiazine tranquilizers (the tranquilizer

Thorazine and related drugs) were introduced. Sometimes, these medications make periods stop.

Rarely, a woman may not menstruate because she has no pituitary gland, either because of surgery, radiation administered to deal with another problem, or as a result of a very severe hemorrhagic shock. In these cases, a woman can usually be helped to ovulate or to menstruate if she wishes.

How do menstrual periods change as a woman gets older?

The number of days a woman with a moderate flow usually has her is period is between five and seven, with more variations in the teen years and in the forties. Almost every woman finds that in her late twenties and early thirties, her periods become shorter and heavier. The day when the flow is heaviest changes, too. When a woman is in her teens and early twenties, the first day is often the heaviest. In her late twenties and early thirties, the morning of the second or third day is usually the heaviest. If she used to bleed for seven days, she may now bleed for five or four. And she may become more regular at this time. In her forties, environmental stress seems to play a bigger part in dictating when a woman menstruates. Periods may show up, for instance, seventeen days after the last one or forty days after the last one. Even if you have been as regular as clockwork, menstruating every twenty-eight days beginning at 11:00 A.M., nothing at all may be wrong when your schedule changes.

What happens if I bleed or spot between periods?

There are three times when women tend to bleed. Many women bleed to some degree at midcycle, when they ovulate. For some, the bleeding is microscopic and goes undetected. Others have as much as a full day of flow. Some have midcycle bleeding from the time they first menstruate. Others begin to have midmonth bleeding in their late thirties and early forties. .

The other two times women frequently bleed are just before or just after their normal period. A number of women with intrauterine birth control devices have brown staining before or after their menstrual flow.

What is important to remember is that bleeding that follows the same pattern month after month is usually fine and healthy; a change in your own personal pattern should send you to your doctor. Random bleeding should always send you for an exam. If you bleed for a day or two, then stop, then bleed again, get a checkup. Polyps, fibroids and other types of tumors cause this kind of bleeding.

Should I expect every period to follow the same pattern of bleeding?

No. In a regularly cycling woman, most periods are nearly identical, but cycles can be thrown off. A period may come early or late, or be skipped entirely. The most common cause is travel. A woman on a business trip may miss her next period; a regularly cycling teen-ager may get no period at all when she is away at camp, then resume menstruating when she returns home. Other women have two groupings of periods. One group is all the same, of equal length and separation. Those are the periods when they ovulate. The other group is made up of periods that are different from the ovulating cycles—coming at different times and lasting a various number of days. These are periods when they haven't ovulated. The length of time between periods and the duration of the bleeding depends on how much uterine lining was built up before the estrogen level dropped. Less lining is built up when ovulation doesn't take place; therefore, these periods are lighter and come earlier then do the others.

How will my period affect any vaginal infection I have?

Women who tend to get monilial vaginitis (*Candida albicans*)—commonly called a fungus or yeast infection—are more likely to get the condition just before or after their periods.

Some of my patients stop using the medications I prescribe to treat these infections, particularly vaginal creams and supposito-

ries, when they menstruate. They should not, and neither should
you unless your physician specifically instructs you to stop.

Can my period cause a vaginal infection to spread to my uterus?

No, vaginal infections do not move up into the uterus. Most vaginal
infections need oxygen, which they get in the vagina. Infections
of the uterus are rare and usually mean something foreign is in that
organ. When I see a uterine infection, also called pelvic inflam-
matory disease (PID), I look for an intrauterine device (IUD), evidence of an incomplete miscarriage or abortion, or venereal disease.

You should suspect a uterine infection if you have tenderness
and pain in the abdomen accompanied by fever. In some instances
there is also some non-period bleeding.

What effect will jogging regularly have on my internal organs or on my period?

Women have been climbing stairs, running after children, jumping
rope, and carrying heavy bundles long distances for centuries, and
not one has had her uterus fall out, yet. Daily jogging should not
cause your internal organs any problems either. If physical work or
exercise really played a role in displacing organs we would see a
lot more written about proper testicular support.

The stress of trying to run a little farther every day, and the loss
of fat, can, make a woman's menstrual cycle irregular. When a
woman takes up running she may change more than her exercise
pattern. Diet and sleep patterns may be altered as well. Her in-
volvement of really "getting into" running can throw her cycle off.

What effect will severe weight swings have on my period?

As I mentioned in Chapter Two, women who lose or gain a lot of
weight often stop menstruating. Every woman needs a minimum
amount of fat in order to cycle, but obese people form a reservoir
of estrogen in their fat cells. The estrogen may not rise and fall

normally. As a result, the woman does not cycle. There are exceptions to the rule, of course. I have patients who weigh 300 pounds and are as regular as clockwork. But a woman of average height (5'3" to 5'5") who gets above 170 or 180 pounds may have period irregularities. Irregularities can also appear in a woman of normal height who drops below 100 pounds.

Is there a physical reason for menstrual cramps?

There is almost always a physical reason for cramps. See Chapter Three for a full explanation.

What does it mean if I am told I have a tipped uterus?

The uterus is not a completely stationary organ. Although it is held in the pelvis by ligaments, the uterus can move forward and backward. Most women (about 60 percent) have uteri shaped like commas, with the top of the organ resting just above the pubic bone. About 25 percent of women's uteri sit straight up and roughly 20 percent have uteri with cervices that face forward, with the rounded tops toward the rear hence "tipped" backward. In the good old days, the tipped uterus was blamed for everything from menstrual cramps to infertility. We now know the tipped uterus is a normal variation.

What is an infantile uterus and what significance does it have?

In a menstruating woman, there is no such thing as an infantile uterus. A small woman may well have a small uterus, but if it's big enough to bleed, it is big enough to get pregnant. And once pregnant, a uterus will grow in size to accommodate the growing fetus.

Does giving birth cure cramps?

It does for some women. Between 30 and 50 percent of women find their cramps diminish or disappear after giving birth. Another third find their cramps are about the same, and about 10 percent have worse cramps after giving birth than they did before.

Does stress cause cramps?

Stress causes the perception of pain to increase at the rate of about 30 percent per hour. General tension and stress, both psychological and physical, make pain feel worse. So if you are worried during this menstrual cycle because, say, your mother is sick, your menstrual cramps are likely to be worse than they were the month before.

Does poor posture cause cramps?

Yes. Cramps in the neck, back, and legs can be caused by poor posture. But cramps in the uterus are not.

Is exercise a surefire solution to cramps?

No. However, it is helpful. Relaxation exercises in particular can enable a woman to cope with the stress with which she usually approaches a painful period. Also, general physical conditioning can help a woman deal with pain. The exercises included in Chapter Five are easy to do and can help you deal with the discomfort.

What effect does an abortion and/or miscarriage have on menstrual cramps?

For most women, probably no effect at all. A few may find that their cramps are less severe afterward.

Why am I the only female in my immediate family with cramps?

A sensitivity to prostaglandins can be genetically transmitted from generation to generation. If your mother and sisters do not have cramps, the tendency may have originated in your father's family.

If your cramps developed years after you started to menstruate, however, you may have secondary dysmenorrhea caused by some physical problem that has developed since you matured. (For more information on secondary dysmenorrhea, see page 35.) It is important to have a physical exam to find out the cause.

What is a D & C (dilation and curettage) and why is one recommended?

D & C stands for dilation and curettage. The cervical opening is stretched with a graduated series of dilating instruments until a small curette (an open, spoon-shaped, sharpened instrument) about a quarter- to a half-inch in diameter can be put into the uterine cavity. The lining of the cavity is then systematically scraped off the uterine wall in a clockwise fashion.

The procedure is recommended for diagnostic reason in cases of abnormal bleeding.

How does a D & C affect menstrual cramps?

The procedure of scraping the inside of the uterus usually doesn't affect cramps and is usually not done to relieve them, although there are women who claim they have gotten relief from the D & C. In the old days, when we had little sense of how small red blood cells are, it was thought a narrow canal increased the pressure inside the uterus and made cramps worse. A D & C, which dilated the canal, would therefore presumably ease the pressure and relieve the pain. But this is untrue. If the blood can get out, the size of the canal is not the cause of cramps.

Very rarely, however, a young woman may have no uterine outlet for the blood and it builds up into a mass in her uterus, causing monthly pain. In this case, her uterus has to be opened up and drained.

How will my mood be affected when I expect my period?

Some women get a little teary right before their periods. One physical cause may be that increased water retention causes the tear ducts to be fuller at that time. I think that women who are slightly depressed get worse before their periods and women who are normally a little anxious get a little more upset.

Can exercise alleviate premenstrual mood swings?

Most people find they are less aware of their irritability if they have a number of specific things to do. Exercise is very useful, not only because of the physical benefits, but because it can be emotionally satisfying. I also tell my patients to make up a list of all the boring tasks they want to get out of the way—jobs such as cleaning out the drawers, washing the kitchen floor, or making a spot inventory check at the office. This time of the month, these tasks can take your mind off your nerves.

Why do female roommates, family members, and office colleagues sometimes menstruate at the same time?

Apparently there are a set of hormones called pheromones that are emitted by the body and picked up by the sense of smell. Some women are thought to be leaders, or "drivers," in establishing menstrual patterns. Their sweat glands emit a kind of signal that programs other women's harmones.

How can I relieve painful premenstrual breast swelling?

Recently, it has been suggested that fluid retention is related to caffeine intake. Some women have had dramatic relief from pain and swelling by cutting caffeine completely out of their diets, or severely limiting their consumption of coffee, cola drinks, chocolate, and anything else they ordinarily consume that contains caffeine.

Any woman who drinks a lot of coffee may have bladder spasms right before menstruating that can be very uncomfortable. Don't forget, too, that caffeine can make you anxious, exacerbating any premenstrual anxieties you may have.

If you retain fluid around the time of your period, try eating a lot of foods rich in potassium, such as dark breads, parsley, spinach, and asparagus. Potassium can help the fluid pass naturally from your system.

Why do I always feel so tired before my period is due?

Many women know they are getting their periods because they feel exhausted. Others don't notice any change at all. The shift in estrogen and progesterone levels have a tiring effect on some. Of course, if you are tired, the best place to go is to bed. But you can also try a dietary approach. Avoid simple carbohydrates (sugars, white bread products): these will make your blood sugar drop two to three hours later, making you feel even more fatigued. A diet full of proteins and complex carbohydrates, such as grains, pastas, and potatoes, will give you more energy for a longer period of time.

Can cramping cause nausea during menstruation or is there a separate reason for queasiness?

The nausea women feel during menstruation is usually a result of the pain. Blood vessels dilate, causing blood pressure to drop, and a woman actually experiences a very mild case of shock. Lying down and putting your feet up will help immensely.

What relation do you see between migraine headaches and the menstrual cycle?

Many women get hormone-related headaches. Others get migraines in a random, stress-related fashion. In women whose migraines only appear at the time of their periods, the prostaglandins produced by the body may be related to spasm of the involuntary muscle in the walls of the arteries, causing pain. In my practice—although not in any controlled, scientific study—I've found some patients get relief from menstrual headaches by taking one of the antiprostaglandins.

Do women on the pill get menstrually-related migraines?

There *are* women taking the birth control pill who get migraine headaches. The estrogen in the pill probably causes spasms in these blood vessels. Women who get headaches should stay away from estrogen, including estrogen replacement therapy during menopause, and the pill because these headaches are precursors of strokes.

Should young women use tampons?

I advise them that it is safest not to. If you can live without using them, do so. We are presently trying to develop a method of absorbing menstrual blood that combines the best of the tampon and the pad, one that conforms to the contours of the body.

Can a tampon get lost in my body?

No. The vagina is a blind pouch, and there is no way a tampon can get lost. But one can get stuck up in the vagina. Or, sometimes a woman will insert a tampon without taking the previous one out. In either case, after a day or two she will get a runny, foul-smelling discharge.

If you can't get a tampon out yourself, call your gynecologist, who should be able to use a speculum and remove it.

Is there a time during the menstrual cycle when women generally feel more sexually aroused?

You can find as many answers to that as there are studies. A good many purport to show that women are more aroused at two different times—at the time of ovulation and during the time they bleed, when coincidentally, many women believe they cannot get pregnant.

What part should tranquilizers play in dealing with anxiety and what cautions should be observed?

Most medical practitioners have become more aware of the side effects of medications and therefore are more sophisticated in dispensing them. Educating the patient in the use of a prescribed drug of any kind is most important. For instance, a woman who is taking tranquilizers because she is tense should know not to mix the drug with alcoholic drinks. That combination is life-threatening. Given adequate diagnosis and monitoring, I see no reason why someone who is very depressed or anxious couldn't take a mild tranquilizer.

How long does it take for your period to resume after you've had an abortion or a baby?

Most women who have had abortions will get their periods in four to eight weeks. The waiting period is about the same after you've had a baby if you don't nurse. If you do nurse, you may get your period after about six months, but it might not come for a year or even longer.

What is toxic shock syndrome (TSS)?

TSS is a rare but serious disease that mostly—but not only—affects menstruating women under the age of thirty who use tampons. Even though only a small number of women have contracted TSS, some of them have died.

The public became aware of toxic shock syndrome in 1980. Little is known about the disease, but current research is generating new information. TSS is thought to be caused by a bacteria called *staphylococcus aureas*, which infects some part of the body, often the vagina, and produces poisons that enter and circulate through the blood stream. The poisons cause various symptoms: a sudden drop in blood pressure that may lead to shock; diarrhea; abdominal tenderness; vomiting; a high fever, at least 102 degrees and very often over 104; and a rash, almost like sunburn, especially on the hands and soles of the feet. The rash is easiest to see on the trunk and neck. It eventually peels.

It is theorized that dry tampons or tampon applicators may cause small cuts or scrapes in the vagina, which in turn may allow bacteria to get into the blood stream. There have been TSS cases in a few women who used sea sponges and diaphragms to collect mentrual fluid; all three internal methods of catching menstrual blood can possibly erode vaginal tissue.

What should I do if I suspect that I have toxic shock?

You should call your doctor immediately or go to the nearest hospital emergency room. Tell them your symptoms and what you suspect you have. Move fast because TSS can rapidly become life-threatening.

If you are using a tampon during your period and you get any of the symptoms, remove the tampon immediately. Don't put in any other internal product until yo have a culture done to see if you have any *Staphylococcus aureas* in your vagina.

Since even a mild case of TSS may create dehydration or very low blood pressure, drink lots of fluids.

Although it is unclear if antibiotics can cure the disease once it has begun, these drugs can lessen the chance of recurrence. Penicillin and ampicillin are no good for this purpose. Antibiotics in the betalactamace antistaphylococcal family are used.

Can men get toxic shock?

Yes. Anyone can if the *Staphylococcus aureas* bacteria gets into the blood stream.

How can you tell if you are hemorrhaging and not just having a heavy period?

If you soak a tampon or pad every ten minutes, you are hemorrhaging. If you soak one every half hour, you are bleeding very heavily; one every hour means you are bleeding heavily.

When you are soaking more than a pad or tampon an hour, you should call your doctor and/or get to a hospital emergency room immediately. Some women have short spates of very heavy bleeding during their periods every month—say, three or four hours. Get to know your own menstrual pattern. Sudden, unexplained bleeding should prompt you to seek medical advise. When you bleed heavily, you should keep your fluid intake high.

Hemorrhage blood is generally brighter and lighter red than regular menstrual blood. The blood gets to where you can see it before it loses its oxygen and the bright color.

What is endometriosis?

Endometriosis is the presence of tissue in the abdominal cavity that would normally be in the lining of the uterus. We don't know why this condition occurs. If those islands of endometrial tissue bleed with each menstrual period, there can be severe pain. Endometriosis can involve enormous tumor masses or tiny nodules. The condition can cause discomfort in some, scarring and infertility in others.

Treatment includes suppressing ovarian function, either with the birth control pill, pregnancy, progesterone, an antihormone drug called Danazol (Danocrine), or surgery to remove the tissue or any scarring.

What are fibroid tumors?

Fibroids are smooth muscle and connective tissue tumors of the uterus, usually in the wall, and sometimes attached to the inside or outside of the uterus by a stalk of connective tissue. They are almost always benign, but may be malignant, especially if they have grown rapidly.

How do fibroid tumors influence menstrual bleeding?

Commonly, they do not. But a fibroid located in the uterine cavity, can increase the surface area of the uterus. Endometrial tissue will cover the fibroid as well as the uterine wall, causing heavy menstrual flow. A fibroid tumor can also cause bleeding at other times. If a fibroid happens to interrupt the normal blood supply to the uterus, it can cause pain off and on at any time of the month.

It is thought that as many as 80 to 90 percent of women develop fibroids. Luckily, they are almost always benign.

How will menopause affect my sex life?

Menopause, just like any other life transition, affects some women positively, a few negatively, and most not at all. A recent study shows 20 percent of the women responding had an increased sex drive and increase in enjoyment, too.

Masters and Johnson's *Human Sexual Response* reports that the amount of vaginal lubrication produced is the same as before menopause; however, the production time is longer. Therefore, it is important that a menopausal woman have adequate foreplay before penetration.

During the reproductive years, estrogen keeps the skin of the vagina thick, like the skin on the palm of your hand. After menopause, vaginal skin is thinner, more like the skin on the back of your hand, and more susceptible to trauma and infection.

All skin is toughened by use. A pregnant woman who expects to nurse is told to toughen her nipples by rubbing them with a rough washcloth. Women who have regular intercourse have an easier time than women whose sex life is interrupted for any length of time by, for example, illness or lack of a partner.

What are hot flashes?

Hot flashes, sometimes called flushes, are wavelike feelings of heat. Most women say they start in the top of the torso and move upward toward the head. Others describe their entire body suddenly getting hot. This feeling of heat is often rapidly followed by copious sweating.

Hot flashes can occur as often as three to five times an hour or as infrequently as once or twice a day. They can stop after a few seconds or, in rare cases, go on for as long as an hour. Only about half the women going through menopause experience them.

How does a hysterectomy affect menopause?

Technically, a hysterectomy is the removal of the uterus, not the estrogen-producing ovaries, and should not affect menopause. If both the ovaries and the uterus are removed in an operation, you go through surgical menopause. Without any estrogen replacement, this menopause is cold turkey, and most women are through with hot flashes and other symptoms in from three to six weeks. A woman who has her uterus removed has no more periods, but she does experience menopausal symptoms whenever her menopause would have occurred naturally, as her ovaries decrease their estrogen production.

Do you recommend estrogen replacement therapy as a solution to menopausal problems?

This is not an easy question to answer. Estrogen is a known carcinogen in humans. It has caused breast cancer in men. It can cause cancer of the uterine lining in women who take it, and cancer of the cervix and vagina in their offspring.

Women may wish to take estrogen to keep their vaginal tissue elastic. Indeed, estrogen is instrumental in thickening the skin of the vagina, as mentioned above. However, the best way to keep vaginal tissues in good shape is to use them. When people's sex lives are interrupted these tissues can deteriorate. Sex is not fun if it hurts, and sometimes a very low oral dosage or a locally applied estrogen cream will relieve the pain. But even a topical application to the vagina will be absorbed into the blood stream.

In general, diet and exercise are far more important than taking estrogen in preventing another menopausal problem: osteoporosis, a condition of reduced bone mass that increases the likelihood of fractures. When demonstrated osteoporosis exists, however, estrogen therapy is often useful and recommended. Anyone taking estrogen therapy should be closely monitored, and seen by a physician at least twice a year.